Slow Cooker

DOG FOOD

The Ultimate Vet-Approved Guide to Well-Balanced, Easy, and Nutritious Homemade Recipes for Your Dog | With Size-Specific Meals, Storage Tips, and Serving Guidelines

MONICA H. PARR

TABLE OF CONTENTS

Chapter 3: 50 Nutritious Recipes for Every Meal

INTRODUCTION

As pet owners, we understand the importance of providing our furry friends with high-quality nutrition to support their health and well-being. With rising concerns about commercial pet food ingredients and processing methods, many dog owners are turning to homemade meals as a healthier alternative. Formed from the foundation of wholesome ingredients packed with essential nutrients and flavor, slow cooking offers a convenient and effective way to prepare healthful meals. Within the pages of this book, nutrition meets companionship, and we offer you a comprehensive guide to preparing nutritious and delicious meals for your canine companion. We'll explore the art and science of slow cooking tailored specifically to meet the dietary needs of dogs. You will learn what sustains our beloved friends and the dedication and care that goes into providing nourishment for our canine companion. In the following chapters, we delve into the fundamentals of slow cooker dog food, from understanding the benefits of this cooking method to selecting the right ingredients and equipment, you'll discover a variety of nutritious recipes crafted with care to ensure optimal canine health and happiness.

Whether you're a seasoned chef wishing to extend your culinary skills or a first-time pet parent looking for advice on providing the finest nutrition for your dog, this book is your go-to guide for producing homemade meals that will keep your canine friend tail-wagging happy and healthy. Join us as we explore culinary creativity and wellness for our canine companion through the slow cooker method.

UNDERSTANDING THE SLOW COOKER APPROACH

Slow cooking has become a popular method in preparing homemade dog meals; it provides various benefits that attend to their nutritional needs and taste preferences. We will learn about all that is involved in the slow cooking approach, stressing its benefits and considerations for preparing wholesome meals that keep your canine companion healthy and satisfied.

Unlike traditional commercial dog foods that may be processed at high temperatures, which can degrade nutrients and alter flavors, slow cooking allows for gentle heating over an extended period. This slow and steady cooking process helps to preserve the nutritional integrity of the ingredients, ensuring that essential vitamins, minerals, and antioxidants remain intact. Slow cooking enhances the flavor and aroma of the ingredients, making the food more appealing to dogs. This can be particularly beneficial for picky eaters or dogs with sensitive appetites, as the rich, savory flavors created during slow cooking can entice them to eat more enthusiastically.

Slow cooking allows for the addition of a wide variety of wholesome ingredients, such as lean meats, fresh vegetables, and whole grains, which provide dogs with a balanced and nutritious diet. By using high-quality, natural ingredients and avoiding artificial additives and preservatives, slow-cooked dog food allows pet owners to experience peace of mind knowing they are providing their companions with wholesome meals free from unnecessary fillers and by-products.

Benefits of Slow Cooking for Dogs

The slow cooking process involves simmering ingredients over low heat for a longer period, allowing different flavors to come together while retaining their nutrients. This mild cooking approach is advantageous for canine nutrition as it preserves the nutrients of the food.

Retained Nutrients

High-temperature cooking methods tend to lead to loss of important micronutrients such as vitamins and minerals but unlike high-temperature cooking methods, slow cooking preserves the nutritional content in the ingredients used while cooking and reduces their exposure to air and water. Since the ingredients are cooked in a sealed pot, this keeps them moist and preserves their nutrients, ensuring your dog receives all the nutrients they need in a balanced proportion. By cooking ingredients at lower temperatures for longer periods, slow cookers or crockpots help maintain the nutritional contents of foods, including proteins, carbohydrates, vitamins, and minerals. This ensures your dog's meals are flavorful and packed with the essential nutrients they need for optimal health and well-being.

Enhanced Digestibility

Foods like meat and vegetables are made up of tough protein fibers and complex sugar structures that are difficult to digest. The lengthy and consistent cooking procedure involved in slow cooking can help break down these compounds. Proteins like collagen and connective tissues are tenderized during the cooking process, and cellulose is broken down into simpler sugar structures, reducing the strain on a dog's digestive tract and allowing the end products of these food compounds to be easily digested. This is particularly beneficial for dogs with sensitive stomachs or difficulties with digestion, senior dogs and dogs with dental issues also benefit from the food derived from the slow cooking process because the softened texture of the food makes it easier to chew and digest. Gastrointestinal upsets or discomforts are less likely to show up because the gentle cooking of slow-cooked meals lowers their possibilities.

Intensified Flavors

Slow cooking allows ingredients to release their natural flavors gradually, producing rich, savory meals that even the most discerning canine palates would love. The slow extraction of aromas increases the anticipation of your dog towards meal time. Allowing flavors to mix over time through slow cooking creates depth in each dish, transforming simple ingredients into culinary delights that your dog will love. Slow-cooked meals create an experience that dogs always find irresistible.

Time Efficiency

While slow cooking requires longer cooking times compared to conventional methods, it offers the convenience of minimal hands-on preparation. Once ingredients are added to the slow cooker, you can set it and forget it, freeing up time for other activities while the meal simmers to perfection. This makes slow cooking an ideal cooking method for busy pet owners who want to provide homemade meals for their dogs without spending hours in the kitchen. With a little planning and preparation, you can have nutritious, homemade dog food ready to serve with minimal effort.

Cost-Effective

Slow cooking enables you to make the most of affordable cuts of meat, seasonal produce, and pantry staples, helping you stretch your pet food budget without compromising on quality. By purchasing ingredients in bulk and utilizing leftovers, you can reduce food waste while providing nutritious meals for your dog. Slow cookers are also energy-efficient appliances that use less electricity than traditional ovens or stovetops, saving you money on your utility bills. With the cost of commercial dog food on the rise, slow cooking offers a budget-friendly alternative that allows you to feed your dog high-quality meals without breaking the bank.

Safety Considerations and Best Practices

While slow cooking offers numerous benefits, it's essential to prioritize safety when preparing homemade meals for your dog. Here are some key considerations and best practices to ensure the health and well-being of your canine companion.

Quality Ingredients

Select high-quality, dog-safe ingredients free from additives, preservatives, and toxic substances. When choosing ingredients for your dog's meals, opt for fresh, whole foods that are free from artificial colors, flavors, and preservatives. Look for ingredients that are sourced from reputable suppliers and labeled as suitable for canine consumption. Avoid processed foods and fillers, such as corn, wheat, and soy, which can be difficult for dogs to digest and may contribute to food allergies or sensitivities.

Proper Handling

Practice proper food safety measures by washing hands, utensils, and surfaces thoroughly before and after handling raw ingredients to prevent cross-contamination and foodborne illness. Keep raw meat and poultry separate from other ingredients to avoid the risk of bacterial contamination. Use separate cutting boards and utensils for raw and cooked foods, and wash them thoroughly with hot, soapy water after each use. Store raw ingredients in the refrigerator at or below 40°F (4°C) to prevent bacterial growth and spoilage. When thawing frozen ingredients, do so in the refrigerator or microwave rather than at room temperature to reduce the risk of bacterial contamination.

Balanced Nutrition

Consult with a veterinarian or canine nutritionist to formulate balanced recipes that meet your dog's specific dietary requirements. Pay attention to the proportions of protein, carbohydrates, fats, vitamins, and minerals in each meal to ensure optimal nutrition. Dogs require a balanced diet that includes a variety of nutrients to support their overall health and well-being. When preparing homemade meals for your dog, aim to include a combination of high-quality proteins, healthy fats, and carbohydrates, as well as essential vitamins and minerals. Choose lean meats, such as chicken, turkey, or beef, as the primary source of protein, and supplement with vegetables, fruits, and whole grains for added nutrition. Avoid feeding your dog exclusively on a single type of food, as this can lead to nutrient deficiencies or imbalances over time.

Safe Cooking Temperatures

Use a food thermometer to monitor cooking temperatures and ensure that meats reach a safe internal temperature of at least 165°F (74°C) to kill harmful bacteria and pathogens. Avoid undercooking meats, poultry, and seafood, as this can increase the risk of foodborne illness in both humans and pets. When using a slow cooker, follow the manufacturer's instructions for cooking times and temperatures, and avoid overfilling the pot to ensure thorough cooking. Use caution when handling hot foods and liquids to prevent burns or scalds and allow cooked meals to cool before serving them to your dog. Be mindful of food safety guidelines when storing leftovers and discard any perishable foods that have been left out at room temperature for more than two hours.

Storage Guidelines

Store cooked meals in airtight containers in the refrigerator for up to three days or freeze in portion-sized servings for longer storage. Label containers with the date and contents for easy identification and use them within the recommended storage time to maintain freshness and quality. When freezing homemade dog food, divide it into individual servings and store them in freezer-safe bags or containers. Thaw frozen meals in the refrigerator overnight or in the microwave on a low setting before serving them to your dog. Avoid refreezing thawed foods, as this can affect their texture and taste. Discard any leftovers that have been thawed but not consumed within 24 hours to prevent bacterial contamination and foodborne illness.

By understanding the benefits of slow cooking and adhering to safety guidelines and best practices, you can provide your dog with homemade meals that are not only nutritious and delicious but also safe and wholesome. Slow cooking offers a convenient and cost-effective way to feed your dog high-quality meals made with fresh, whole ingredients. If you're cooking for a healthy adult dog or a senior dog with special dietary needs, slow cooker dog food can be tailored to meet their individual needs. With a little time and effort, you can create homemade meals that nourish your dog's body and soul, strengthening the bond between you and them.

Chapter 1

THE BASICS OF
SLOW COOKER
DOG FOOD

The fundamentals of preparing homemade dog food involve a careful balance of certain principles to make sure your furry friend receives a nutritious and well-rounded diet tailored to their individual needs.

First and foremost, consulting with your veterinarian is important before making any dietary changes for your dog. Your vet can provide valuable insights into your dog's specific nutritional requirements based on factors such as age, breed, weight, and any existing health conditions. With this information, you can now go ahead to prepare homemade meals using the slow cooker method that caters to your dog's unique needs.

At the heart of homemade dog food is balanced nutrition; just like humans, dogs require a mix of protein, carbohydrates, fats, vitamins, and minerals to thrive. Protein serves as the building blocks for your dog's muscles, organs, and tissues, so it's crucial to include high-quality sources in their diet. Lean meats such as chicken, turkey, beef, and fish are excellent choices, providing essential amino acids for your dog's overall health. However, the protein content should be adjusted to your dog's requirements, considering factors like age, activity level, and health status.

Another macronutrient, carbohydrate, plays a vital role in your dog's energy levels and digestive health. Whole grains like brown rice, oats, and quinoa are nutritious sources of carbohydrates, offering fiber and energy to boost your dog's daily activities. Starchy vegetables such as sweet potatoes and pumpkin are also valuable carbohydrate sources, providing vitamins, minerals, and antioxidants. When preparing homemade dog food, aim for a balanced mix of proteins, carbohydrates, and fats to meet your dog's nutritional needs.

Healthy fats are essential for your dog's skin, coat, and overall well-being. Adding healthy fat to your canine diet can help maintain your dog's skin and coat health while supporting their immune system. However, try to avoid excessive amounts of saturated fats or unhealthy oils, which can lead to weight gain and other health issues. Be mindful of the fat content in your dog's diet and opt for healthier sources to promote their overall health.

In addition to macronutrients like protein, carbohydrates, and fats, homemade dog food should also include a variety of micronutrients to ensure your dog receives all the essential vitamins and minerals they need to thrive. Vegetables and fruits are excellent sources of vitamins, minerals, and antioxidants, providing valuable nutrients to support your dog's immune system and overall health. Carrots, broccoli, spinach, blueberries, and apples are just a few examples of dog-safe fruits and vegetables that can be incorporated into homemade meals. However, it's essential to cook or finely chop these ingredients to aid in digestion and help nutrient absorption. Calcium is another essential nutrient that should be included in homemade dog food to support bone health and muscle function. If your homemade dog food recipe does not include an organic calcium source like cheese, you may need to supplement it with calcium to ensure your dog receives an adequate amount.

Other supplements such as vitamin and mineral blends may be necessary to fill any nutritional gaps in your dog's diet. Consult with your veterinarian to determine the right supplements for your dog's specific needs. Portion control is crucial when preparing homemade dog food to prevent overfeeding or underfeeding. Follow feeding guidelines provided by your veterinarian and adjust portion sizes based on your dog's weight, activity level, and body condition. Be sure to monitor your dog's weight regularly and make adjustments to their diet as needed to maintain a healthy weight and body condition.

Food safety is paramount when preparing homemade dog food to prevent contamination and ensure your dog's well-being. Cook meats thoroughly to kill any harmful bacteria, handle ingredients safely to avoid cross-contamination, and store leftovers properly in the refrigerator or freezer to prevent spoilage. By practicing good food safety habits, you can mitigate the risk of foodborne illnesses and keep your dog safe and healthy. If you're transitioning your dog from commercial dog food to homemade meals, it's essential to do so gradually over several days to allow your dog's digestive system to adjust. Start by mixing small amounts of homemade food with their regular diet and gradually increase the proportion of homemade food while decreasing the commercial food. Monitor your dog's response to the transition and make any necessary adjustments to ensure a smooth transition to their new diet.

SELECTING QUALITY INGREDIENTS

The foundation of any nutritious dog food recipe begins with high-quality ingredients. When shopping for ingredients for your slow cooker dog food recipes, prioritize fresh, whole foods that are free from additives, preservatives, and toxic substances. Look for lean cuts of meat, such as chicken, turkey, beef, or lamb, as the primary protein source. Go for organic options whenever possible to ensure the highest quality and nutritional value.

In addition to protein, include a variety of vegetables and fruits in your dog's meals to provide essential vitamins, minerals, and antioxidants. Carrots, sweet potatoes, peas, spinach, and blueberries are excellent choices that offer a range of health benefits for dogs. Be sure to wash and chop vegetables and fruits into small, bite-sized pieces to make them easier for your dog to digest.

When it comes to carbohydrates, choose whole grains such as brown rice, quinoa, oats, or barley. These grains provide a source of energy and fiber, helping to support digestive health and maintain stable blood sugar levels in dogs. Avoid refined grains and gluten-containing ingredients, as these can be difficult for dogs to digest and may contribute to food sensitivities or allergies. It is also important to note that dogs are carnivores so recipes must contain fewer grains as an ingredient.

Quality Ingredients in Canine Nutrition

Protein Sources

1. **Chicken:** Lean protein source that is easy to digest and versatile in dog food recipes.
2. **Turkey:** Another lean protein that is hypoallergenic and suitable for dogs with food sensitivities.
3. **Beef:** Rich in essential amino acids, iron, and vitamins, making it a great protein source.
4. **Lamb:** Good for dogs with food allergies, high in protein and essential fatty acids.
5. **Fish (e.g., Haddock, trout, cod):** High in omega-3 fatty acids, which promote a healthy coat and reduce inflammation.
6. **Eggs:** Excellent source of protein, vitamins, and minerals. They also contain healthy fats.

7. **Duck:** Rich in iron and amino acids, and a good alternative protein for dogs with allergies.
8. **Venison:** Lean protein that is less likely to cause allergies, rich in nutrients.
9. **Rabbit:** Lean protein with a high content of essential amino acids and minerals.

Carbohydrate Sources

1. **Brown Rice:** High in fiber and provides a good source of energy.
2. **Oats:** Easy to digest and good for dogs with wheat allergies.
3. **Barley:** High in fiber and good for digestive health.
4. **Sweet Potatoes:** Rich in vitamins A and C, and a good source of dietary fiber.
5. **Quinoa:** Complete protein source that is gluten-free and highly nutritious.
6. **Pumpkin:** High in fiber and beta-carotene, beneficial for digestive health.
7. **Butternut Squash:** Rich in vitamins and minerals, and good for digestive health.
8. **Lentils:** High in protein and fiber, making them a good plant-based protein source.
9. **Chickpeas:** High in protein, fiber, and vitamins, and good for heart health.
10. **Peas:** Rich in protein, fiber, and vitamins, and beneficial for overall health.

Fat And Oil Sources

1. **Fish Oil (e.g., cod liver oil):** Rich in omega-3 fatty acids, which promote a healthy coat and reduce inflammation.
2. **Flaxseed Oil:** Good source of omega-3 and omega-6 fatty acids, which support skin and coat health.
3. **Coconut Oil:** Contains medium-chain triglycerides (MCTs) that can boost energy and support cognitive function.
4. **Chicken Fat:** High in essential fatty acids and palatability, enhancing the flavor of dog food.
5. **Olive Oil:** Good source of monounsaturated fats and antioxidants, supporting overall health.

Fruit Sources

1. **Blueberries:** High in antioxidants, vitamins, and fiber, beneficial for immune health.
2. **Apples (without seeds):** Good source of vitamins A and C, and fiber, supporting digestive health.
3. **Bananas:** Rich in potassium and vitamins, providing a quick source of energy.
4. **Strawberries:** High in antioxidants and vitamins, promoting overall health.

5. **Cranberries:** Good for urinary tract health and rich in antioxidants.
6. **Watermelon (without seeds):** Hydrating and rich in vitamins A, B6, and C.
7. **Pears (without seeds):** High in fiber and vitamins, good for digestive health.
8. **Mango (without pit):** Rich in vitamins A, B6, C, and E, and beneficial for immune health.
9. **Pineapple:** Contains bromelain, which aids digestion and is rich in vitamins.
10. **Peaches (without pit):** Good source of fiber and vitamins A and C.

Vegetable Sources

1. **Carrots:** High in beta-carotene, fiber, and vitamins, promoting eye health and digestion.
2. **Green Beans:** Low in calories and high in fiber, good for weight management.
3. **Spinach:** Rich in vitamins A, C, and K, and minerals like iron and calcium.
4. **Broccoli:** High in fiber, vitamins, and antioxidants, supporting overall health.
5. **Kale:** Nutrient-dense leafy green, rich in vitamins A, C, and K, and antioxidants.
6. **Zucchini:** Low in calories and high in fiber, good for digestive health.
7. **Celery:** Low in calories and rich in vitamins and minerals, promoting overall health.
8. **Cauliflower:** High in fiber and vitamins, supporting digestive and immune health.
9. **Bell Peppers:** Rich in vitamins A and C, and antioxidants, supporting immune health.
10. **Cucumber:** Hydrating and low in calories, good for weight management.

UNDERSTANDING CANINE NUTRITIONAL NEEDS

To create balanced and nutritious meals for your dog, it's essential to understand their specific nutritional requirements. Dogs are omnivores with dietary needs that differ from humans, requiring a diet that is rich in protein, moderate in fat, and low in carbohydrates. Protein is essential for building and repairing tissues, supporting muscle growth, and maintaining a healthy immune system in dogs.

In addition to protein, dogs require essential fatty acids, vitamins, and minerals to support overall health and well-being. Omega-3 and omega-6 fatty acids are particularly important for maintaining healthy skin and coat, reducing inflammation, and supporting brain function in dogs. Vitamins such as A, D, E, and B-complex vitamins play crucial roles in metabolism, immune function, and cell growth and repair. Minerals such as calcium, phosphorus, potassium, and magnesium are also essential for maintaining strong bones, teeth, and muscles in dogs.

It's important to strike the right balance of nutrients in your dog's meals to prevent deficiencies or imbalances that can negatively impact their health. Consult with a veterinarian or canine nutritionist to ensure that your homemade dog food recipes meet your dog's specific nutritional needs based on factors such as age, breed, size, and activity level.

BALANCING MACRONUTRIENTS IN HOMEMADE MEALS

The percentages of macronutrients that make up the total calories in a dog's diet are:

- **Proteins:** 50-75%
- **Carbohydrates:** 15-35%
- **Fats:** 10-15%

Achieving the right balance of macronutrients – protein, fat, and carbohydrates – is crucial for creating homemade dog food that meets your dog's nutritional requirements. Protein should make up the majority of your dog's diet, comprising approximately 50-75% of total calories. Choose high-quality protein sources such as meat, poultry, fish, eggs, and dairy products to provide essential amino acids for muscle growth and repair.

Fat is another important macronutrient that provides a concentrated source of energy for dogs. Aim to include healthy fats from sources such as lean meats, fish oil, flaxseed oil, and coconut oil in your dog's meals, achieving between 10-15%. Limit saturated fats and avoid trans fats, as these can contribute to obesity, heart disease, and other health problems in dogs.

Carbohydrates should make up the remaining portion of your dog's diet, comprising approximately 25-50% of total calories. Choose complex carbohydrates such as whole grains, legumes, and starchy vegetables to provide sustained energy and dietary fiber for digestive health. Avoid simple carbohydrates and refined sugars, as these can cause spikes in blood sugar levels and contribute to weight gain and insulin resistance in dogs.

FORBIDDEN FOODS IN CANINE NUTRITION

While many foods are safe and beneficial for dogs, several foods should be avoided due to their potential toxicity or harmful effects on canine health. These forbidden foods include:

Chocolate

Chocolate is harmful to dogs primarily due to its content of theobromine and caffeine, both of which are toxic to canines. Theobromine, in particular, is metabolized slowly in dogs compared to humans, leading to a buildup of the toxin in their system. Even small amounts of chocolate can cause toxicity in dogs, affecting their central nervous system and cardiovascular system. Symptoms of chocolate poisoning include increased heart rate, agitation, tremors, seizures, vomiting, diarrhea, and rapid breathing. The severity of chocolate toxicity depends on factors such as the type of chocolate ingested, the dog's size and weight, and their sensitivity to theobromine. Dark chocolate and unsweetened baking chocolate contain higher concentrations of theobromine compared to milk chocolate or white chocolate, making them more toxic to dogs. Dog owners must keep all chocolate products out of reach of their pets

Grapes and Raisins

Grapes and raisins are toxic to dogs, although the exact compound responsible for their toxicity is not yet identified. Even small amounts of grapes or raisins can cause severe kidney damage in dogs, leading to symptoms such as vomiting, diarrhea, lethargy, decreased appetite, abdominal pain, and increased thirst and urination. In some cases, ingestion of grapes or raisins can lead to kidney failure and even death. The toxic effects of grapes and raisins can occur regardless of the dog's size, breed, or age, and there is currently no known safe threshold for consumption. As a result, dog owners need to avoid feeding grapes, raisins, or any products containing these fruits to their pets. If a dog ingests grapes or raisins, immediate veterinary attention is necessary to initiate treatment and reduce the risk of kidney damage or other complications.

Onions and Garlic

Onions and garlic are harmful to dogs because they contain compounds called thiosulfates and disulfides, which can cause oxidative damage to a dog's red blood cells, leading to a condition known as hemolytic anemia. Hemolytic anemia results in the destruction of red blood cells, impairing the body's ability to transport oxygen to tissues and organs. Even small amounts of onions or garlic, whether raw, cooked, or powdered, can be toxic to dogs. Symptoms of onion or garlic poisoning in dogs may include weakness, lethargy, pale gums, rapid breathing, vomiting, diarrhea, abdominal pain, and dark urine. In severe cases, ingestion of onions or garlic can lead to collapse, organ damage, and even death. Dog owners need to avoid feeding their pets any foods containing onions, garlic, or related ingredients, such as onion powder or garlic powder. This includes common human foods like onion rings, garlic bread, and certain sauces or seasonings. Additionally, be cautious when feeding dogs leftovers or table scraps, as these may contain onion or garlic ingredients.

Xylitol

Xylitol is a sugar alcohol commonly used as a sugar substitute in many products, including sugar-free gum, candies, baked goods, toothpaste, and certain medications. While xylitol is safe for humans, it can be highly toxic to dogs. When dogs ingest xylitol, it causes a rapid release of insulin from the pancreas, leading to a sudden and severe decrease in blood sugar levels, known as hypoglycemia. Hypoglycemia can result in symptoms such as weakness, lethargy, disorientation, seizures, collapse, and even death if left untreated. Additionally, xylitol can also cause liver damage and failure in dogs, even at lower doses. The toxic effects of xylitol can occur within minutes to hours after ingestion, depending on the amount consumed and the size of the dog. Even small amounts of xylitol can be dangerous, and the severity of toxicity can vary depending on factors such as the dog's size, breed, and overall health. It's essential for dog owners to be vigilant about the presence of xylitol in their homes and to keep all products containing xylitol out of reach of their pets. This includes checking ingredient labels carefully, especially on sugar-free products, gums, candies, and medications. If you suspect your dog has ingested xylitol, seek immediate veterinary attention, even if your dog appears asymptomatic, as prompt treatment is crucial to prevent potentially life-threatening complications.

Alcohol

Alcohol is toxic to dogs and can have severe and potentially life-threatening effects on their health. The main reason alcohol is harmful to dogs is that their bodies process it differently than humans. Dogs are much more sensitive to alcohol's effects due to their smaller size and different metabolism. When dogs ingest alcohol, it quickly gets absorbed into their bloodstream, leading to symptoms of intoxication. These symptoms can include disorientation, lethargy, vomiting, diarrhea, loss of coordination, difficulty breathing, and even seizures or coma in severe cases. Additionally, alcohol can depress a dog's central nervous system, leading to respiratory depression and a drop in blood pressure. Even small amounts of alcohol can be dangerous for dogs, and ingestion of large quantities can be fatal. The toxic effects of alcohol can occur rapidly, and immediate veterinary attention is necessary if you suspect your dog has ingested any alcohol. Dog owners must keep all alcoholic beverages, including beer, wine, liquor, and cocktails, out of reach of their pets. Additionally, be mindful of other products that may contain alcohol, such as certain medications, mouthwashes, and household cleaning products. Always store these items securely and be cautious when using them around pets.

Avocado

Avocado contains a substance called a fungicidal toxin called persin, which can be toxic to dogs in certain circumstances. While the persin content in ripe avocado fruit is relatively low and typically not harmful to dogs in small amounts, other parts of the avocado plant, such as the leaves, bark, and pit (seed), contain higher concentrations of persin and can be more toxic. Ingestion of large quantities of avocado, including the pit and skin, can potentially lead to gastrointestinal upset in dogs, such as vomiting and diarrhea. Additionally, the high-fat content in avocado can cause pancreatitis, a painful and potentially serious inflammation of the pancreas, especially in dogs with underlying health conditions or those prone to digestive issues. Furthermore, the avocado pit poses a choking hazard and can cause an intestinal obstruction if ingested by dogs, leading to abdominal discomfort, vomiting, and potentially requiring surgical intervention to remove. While small amounts of ripe avocado flesh are generally considered safe for most dogs, it's best to err on the side of caution and avoid feeding avocado products to dogs altogether, especially in large quantities or if they have a history of gastrointestinal sensitivity. If your dog accidentally ingests avocado or shows any signs of illness after consuming it, consult your veterinarian for guidance and appropriate treatment.

Macadamia Nuts

Macadamia nuts are highly toxic to dogs and can cause a range of symptoms when ingested, even in small amounts. The exact mechanism of toxicity is not fully understood, but even a small number of macadamia nuts can lead to significant health problems in dogs. When dogs consume macadamia nuts, they can experience symptoms such as weakness, lethargy, vomiting, tremors, difficulty walking, muscle stiffness, joint pain, and an elevated body temperature. These symptoms typically occur within 12 hours of ingestion and can last for up to 48 hours or more. The exact compound or compounds in macadamia nuts responsible for their toxicity to dogs are not yet identified, but even small quantities of these nuts can cause adverse effects. Additionally, the specific sensitivity to macadamia nuts varies among individual dogs, with some dogs experiencing more severe symptoms than others. It's essential for dog owners to be aware of the dangers of macadamia nuts and to keep all products containing these nuts out of reach of their pets. This includes not only whole macadamia nuts but also products containing macadamia nuts, such as cookies, candies, and trail mixes.

Bones

Bones, often seen as a natural treat for dogs, can pose several risks to their health. One of the most significant dangers is the potential for bones to splinter, especially cooked bones, which can lead to sharp fragments causing lacerations or puncture wounds in a dog's mouth, throat, or digestive tract. Additionally, bones can present a choking hazard, particularly if they are small or irregularly shaped. Ingestion of bones, whether whole or in fragments, can also lead to digestive issues such as constipation, diarrhea, or gastrointestinal blockages. Furthermore, chewing on hard bones can cause dental damage, including fractured teeth or gum injuries. While bones contain some nutrients, they are not a complete or balanced source of nutrition for dogs, and feeding bones as a regular part of a dog's diet can lead to nutritional imbalances and deficiencies over time. Moreover, raw bones may harbor harmful bacteria such as Salmonella or E. coli, posing a risk of foodborne illness to both dogs and their owners. Considering these potential risks, it's essential for dog owners to be cautious when offering bones to their pets and to consider safer alternatives such as specially designed chew toys or dental treats that promote dental health and satisfy a dog's natural urge to chew.

Raw Dough

Raw dough poses significant risks to dogs due to its yeast and raw flour content. When ingested, the warmth and moisture in a dog's stomach create an ideal environment for the yeast to ferment, causing the dough to expand and rise. This expansion can lead to gastric distension, where the stomach becomes bloated and uncomfortable. In severe cases, gastric distension can progress to Gastric Dilatation and Volvulus (GDV), a life-threatening condition where the stomach twists upon itself, trapping gas and causing severe abdominal pain and potential organ damage. Additionally, yeast fermentation produces alcohol as a byproduct, leading to alcohol poisoning in dogs. Raw flour, another component of raw dough, may contain harmful bacteria such as E. coli or Salmonella, posing a risk of foodborne illness and gastrointestinal upset. Furthermore, raw dough lacks essential nutrients and can lead to nutritional imbalances if ingested regularly. To prevent these risks, dog owners should keep baking ingredients out of reach of their pets and seek immediate veterinary attention if their dog ingests raw dough or displays any signs of distress afterward. Early intervention will reduce the risk of complications and ensure the dog's well-being.

Moldy or Spoiled Foods

Moldy or spoiled foods are harmful to dogs because they can contain toxins produced by mold or harmful bacteria that can cause a range of health problems. When dogs ingest moldy or spoiled foods, they may be exposed to toxins such as mycotoxins and aflatoxins produced by certain types of mold, which can lead to poisoning and adverse health effects. Additionally, spoiled foods may harbor harmful bacteria such as Salmonella, E. coli, or Listeria, which can cause foodborne illnesses in dogs, leading to symptoms such as vomiting, diarrhea, abdominal pain, fever, and lethargy. In severe cases, ingestion of moldy or spoiled foods can result in more serious complications, including neurological problems and organ damage or failure. To prevent these risks, it's essential for dog owners to properly store and handle food, promptly discard any moldy or spoiled foods, and supervise their pets to prevent access to potentially harmful substances. If a dog ingests moldy or spoiled food or shows any signs of illness afterward.

Caffeine

Caffeine is harmful to dogs because they are much more sensitive to its effects compared to humans. Dogs metabolize caffeine more slowly, leading to a buildup of the stimulant in their system, which can have toxic effects. Caffeine stimulates the central nervous system and can lead to symptoms such as restlessness, agitation, rapid breathing, tremors, elevated heart rate, hypertension (high blood pressure), seizures, and even death in severe cases. The amount of caffeine required to cause toxicity in dogs varies depending on factors such as the dog's size, breed, age, and individual sensitivity. However, even small amounts of caffeine can be dangerous for dogs, especially those with preexisting health conditions or those who accidentally ingest caffeine-containing products. Caffeine is commonly found in coffee, tea, energy drinks, soda, chocolate, certain medications (such as cold and flu remedies, pain relievers, and weight loss supplements), and other products. Dog owners should be vigilant about keeping these items out of reach of their pets to prevent accidental ingestion.

Understanding the basics of slow cooker dog food, including selecting quality ingredients, understanding canine nutritional needs, balancing macronutrients, and avoiding forbidden foods, is essential in creating balanced and nutritious meals that support your dog's health and well-being. Also, note that it is crucial to seek veterinary attention promptly to address any potential health concerns and ensure the best possible outcome for the dog's health.

Chapter 2

ESSENTIAL EQUIPMENT AND PREPARATION

Introducing slow cooker dog food into your pet's diet requires special equipment and thorough preparation to ensure the meals are nutritious and safe. At the core of your kitchen arsenal is a reliable slow cooker, chosen in a size suitable for your dog's portion sizes and equipped with features like programmable settings for convenience. Gathering high-quality ingredients is crucial, including lean proteins like chicken, turkey, or fish, wholesome carbohydrates such as brown rice or sweet potatoes, and a variety of dog-safe vegetables and fruits, all free from harmful additives or seasonings. A sturdy cutting board and a sharp knife are essential for chopping ingredients, while accurate measuring utensils ensure balanced nutrition in your dog's meals. Consider using homemade or low-sodium store-bought stock or broth as a flavorful liquid base and prepare storage containers for portioning and storing the cooked food. Consulting with your veterinarian before starting is vital to ensure the recipes align with your dog's dietary needs and health requirements, providing valuable guidance for a successful transition to slow cooker dog food. With the right equipment, ingredients, and professional advice, you can create delicious and nutritious meals tailored to your dog's well-being and enjoyment.

In this chapter, we'll explore the essential equipment and preparation techniques necessary for successful slow cooker dog food. From choosing the right slow cooker to preparing ingredients and tips for successful cooking, we'll cover everything you need to know to get started on your homemade dog food journey.

CHOOSING THE RIGHT SLOW COOKER

The slow cooker, also known as a crock pot, is a versatile kitchen appliance that allows for convenient and hands-free cooking of soups, stews, and other dishes. When selecting a slow cooker for preparing dog food, several considerations ensure you choose the most suitable option. Begin by assessing the size of your dog and the amount of food you plan to prepare, opting for a slow cooker with a capacity that aligns with your needs. Features such as programmable settings, digital timers, and automatic warming functions enhance convenience and versatility, allowing precise control over cooking times and temperatures. Lay emphasis on materials that are durable, easy to clean, and safe for food preparation, such as models with dishwasher-safe ceramic or stoneware inserts. The shape also plays a role, with oval-shaped slow cookers ideal for larger cuts of meat and round-shaped ones offering versatility for various recipes. Factor in your budget while considering safety features like cool-touch handles and secure lids to prevent accidents. Researching reviews and ratings provides valuable insights into performance and user satisfaction, helping you make an informed decision. Choosing the right slow cooker involves the listed considerations:

Size

The size of a slow cooker significantly influences the preparation and outcome of your dog's meals. A larger slow cooker allows for the preparation of more substantial batches of dog food, making it suitable for households with multiple dogs or for those who prefer batch cooking for convenience. With a larger capacity, you can cook larger portions of food in a single session, reducing the need for frequent cooking and allowing for efficient meal preparation, particularly for busy pet owners. Additionally, a larger slow cooker offers greater flexibility in adapting recipes or experimenting with different ingredients, providing ample space to accommodate various flavors and textures. However, smaller slow cookers may be sufficient for smaller dogs or for those who prefer to cook single servings or smaller batches at a time. Choose a slow cooker size that accommodates the amount of food you plan to prepare for your dog. For small to medium-sized dogs, a **4- to 6-quart** slow cooker is typically sufficient, while larger dogs may require a **6- to 8-quart** model.

Temperature Settings

The temperature settings of a slow cooker play a crucial role in determining its suitability for preparing dog meals, influencing cooking times, food safety, and flavor development. When choosing a slow cooker for dog meals, it's essential to consider the temperature settings available and how they align with your cooking preferences and the ingredients you plan to use. Most slow cookers offer low, high, and sometimes medium temperature settings, allowing for flexibility in cooking a variety of recipes. Low-temperature settings are ideal for slow and gentle cooking over an extended period, which is often preferred for preparing dog meals as it helps retain nutrients and flavors while breaking down tough ingredients like meats and vegetables. This low and slow cooking method also ensures thorough cooking and food safety, especially when using raw ingredients. High-temperature settings, on the other hand, provide faster cooking times and are suitable for recipes that require quicker preparation, such as heating pre-cooked ingredients or reducing cooking times for certain dishes. However, high temperatures may lead to overcooking or drying out of ingredients, so they should be used cautiously for dog meals to avoid compromising texture and flavor. Additionally, some slow cookers offer programmable temperature settings or features like a keep-warm function, allowing for greater control in meal preparation.

Shape

Slow cookers come in various shapes, including round and oval, each with its advantages and considerations. Round slow cookers are more versatile and suitable for a wide range of recipes, making them a popular choice for many households. They evenly distribute heat and are ideal for cooking stews, soups, and sauces, as well as for braising meats or cooking grains and legumes. However, round slow cookers may have limited space for larger cuts of meat or whole poultry, requiring them to be cut into smaller pieces to fit comfortably. On the other hand, oval slow cookers have a longer, more elongated shape, providing ample space for larger cuts of meat and whole poultry without the need for cutting. This makes them ideal for preparing roasts, whole chickens, or other large cuts of meat for your dog's meals. Additionally, the elongated shape allows for better distribution of ingredients, ensuring even cooking and thorough flavor development. When choosing a slow cooker for dog meals, consider the types of recipes you plan to prepare and whether a round or oval shape would better suit your cooking needs and preferences.

Features

The features of a slow cooker play a vital role in determining its suitability for preparing dog meals, offering convenience, versatility, and safety features that can enhance the cooking experience. When choosing a slow cooker for dog meals, consider features such as programmable settings, timers, automatic warming functions, and removable inserts. Programmable settings allow you to customize cooking times and temperatures according to your recipe's requirements, providing flexibility and precision in meal preparation. Timers ensure precise cooking and prevent overcooking, allowing you to set the slow cooker to start cooking at a specific time and finish cooking when you're ready to serve the meal. Automatic warming functions keep food warm after cooking, ideal for busy schedules or when preparing meals in advance, ensuring that your dog's food remains fresh and ready to serve whenever needed, and removable inserts make it easier to clean. Safety features such as cool-touch handles, secure locking lids, and stable, non-slip bases help prevent accidents and injuries while handling the slow cooker, providing a safe cooking environment.

PREPARING INGREDIENTS FOR SLOW COOKING

Before adding ingredients to your slow cooker, it's essential to prepare them properly to ensure optimal flavor and texture. Follow these steps to prepare ingredients for slow cooking.

Meat

1. **Trim Excess Fat:** Start by trimming any visible fat from the meat and poultry using a sharp knife. Excess fat can contribute to a greasy texture in the final dish and may be difficult for your dog to digest. Removing fat also helps reduce the overall calorie content of the meal.

2. **Brown Meats (Optional):** While not strictly necessary, browning meats in a skillet before adding them to the slow cooker can enhance their flavor and texture. Heat a skillet over medium heat and add a small amount of oil or cooking spray. Once hot, add the meat in batches, ensuring that each piece has enough space to brown evenly. Cook until the meat develops a golden-brown crust on all sides, then transfer it to the slow cooker. Browning meat caramelizes its surface, resulting in richer flavors and a more appealing appearance in the finished dish.

Vegetables

1. **Wash Thoroughly:** Rinse vegetables under cold running water to remove any dirt, debris, or pesticides. Use a vegetable brush or scrubber to gently clean the surface of root vegetables like carrots and potatoes. Washing vegetables helps remove contaminants and ensures that they are safe for consumption.

2. **Chop Into Bite-Sized Pieces:** Use a sharp knife to chop vegetables into uniform, bite-sized pieces. This not only ensures even cooking but also makes it easier for your dog to eat and digest. Remove any seeds, pits, or stems that may be harmful to dogs, such as apple seeds, cherry pits, or tomato stems.

3. **Steam or Blanch (Optional):** While some vegetables can be added directly to the slow cooker, others may benefit from pre-cooking to soften their texture and enhance their flavor. Steam or blanch vegetables like carrots, sweet potatoes, and green beans before adding them to the slow cooker. To steam, place the vegetables in a steamer basket over boiling water and cook until tender. To blanch, immerse the vegetables in boiling water for a few minutes, and then transfer them to an ice bath to stop the cooking process. Pre-cooking vegetables can also help retain their vibrant color and nutrients.

Grains

1. **Rinse Thoroughly:** Rinse grains such as rice, quinoa, or barley under cold running water to remove excess starch and debris. This helps prevent grains from becoming overly sticky or gummy during cooking and ensures a light and fluffy texture in the finished dish.

2. **Use Whole Grains:** Opt for whole grains rather than refined grains to provide your dog with added fiber, vitamins, and minerals. Whole grains are less processed and retain more of their natural nutrients, making them a healthier choice for your dog's diet. Common whole grains include brown rice, quinoa, oats, and barley.

Liquids

1. **Add Flavorful Broth:** Enhance the flavor of your slow cooker meals by adding broth, water, or other liquid ingredients to create a flavorful cooking base. Choose low-sodium broth or homemade bone broth to control the sodium content of your dog's meals and avoid excessive salt intake. Homemade broth is particularly beneficial as it allows you to control the ingredients and avoid additives or preservatives commonly found in store-bought varieties.

2. **Control Sodium Intake:** Be mindful of the sodium content in broth and other liquid ingredients, as excessive salt intake can lead to health issues such as high blood pressure and kidney problems in dogs. Opt for low-sodium options whenever possible and avoid adding additional salt or salty seasonings to your dog's meals.

Beans and Legumes

1. **Soak Overnight (Optional):** If using dried beans or legumes such as kidney beans, lentils, or chickpeas, consider soaking them overnight before cooking. Soaking helps soften the beans, reduce cooking time, and improve digestibility. Rinse the soaked beans thoroughly before adding them to the slow cooker.

2. **Cook Beans Separately:** Some beans, such as kidney beans, contain naturally occurring toxins that can be harmful if not properly cooked. To ensure safety, cook beans separately in boiling water for at least 10 minutes before adding them to the slow cooker. Discard the cooking water and rinse the beans before adding them to your recipe.

3. **Use Canned Beans (Optional):** For added convenience, you can use canned beans instead of dried beans. Be sure to rinse canned beans thoroughly under cold running water to remove excess salt and preservatives before adding them to the slow cooker. Canned beans are pre-cooked and require less cooking time than dried beans.

Fruits

1. **Peel and Remove Seeds:** When using fruits such as apples, pears, or peaches in slow cooker recipes, peel them and remove any seeds, pits, or cores that may be harmful to dogs. Seeds and pits contain compounds that can be toxic or pose a choking hazard, so it's essential to remove them before cooking.

2. **Chop Into Small Pieces:** Chop fruits into small, bite-sized pieces to make them easier for your dog to eat and digest. Remove any tough or fibrous parts, such as apple cores or peach pits that may be difficult for your dog to chew.

3. **Add Citrus Zest (Optional):** For added flavor, you can add citrus zest from fruits such as oranges, lemons, or limes to your slow cooker recipes. Citrus zest contains aromatic oils that can enhance the taste of your dog's meals without adding extra calories or sodium. Be sure to use organic citrus fruits and wash them thoroughly before zesting to remove any pesticides or wax.

Herbs and Spices

1. **Choose Dog-Safe Herbs:** When seasoning your dog's meals, opt for dog-safe herbs and spices that are free from toxic compounds and additives. Some safe options include parsley, basil, oregano, thyme, and rosemary. Avoid using onions, garlic, chives, and other members of the allium family, as these can be harmful to dogs in large quantities.

2. **Use Fresh or Dried Herbs:** You can use fresh or dried herbs to season your dog's meals, depending on your preference and availability. Fresh herbs have a more vibrant flavor and aroma but may spoil more quickly, while dried herbs have a longer shelf life but may be less potent.

3. **Crush or Chop Herbs (Optional):** To release their flavors and aromas, crush or chop fresh herbs before adding them to your slow cooker recipes. This helps ensure that the herbs are evenly distributed throughout the dish and infuse the food with their delicious flavors.

TIPS FOR SUCCESSFUL SLOW COOKING

The tips offered in this section ensure successful slow cooking and delicious.

Layer Ingredients

1. **Distribute Evenly:** When layering ingredients in the slow cooker, aim to distribute them evenly to promote uniform cooking. Spread meat and dense vegetables evenly across the bottom of the slow cooker to ensure they receive ample heat and cook thoroughly.

2. **Create Layers:** Layer ingredients in the slow cooker, starting with protein-rich foods like meat or poultry, followed by denser vegetables such as carrots or potatoes, and finishing with softer vegetables and grains on top. This layering technique helps ensure that all ingredients cook evenly and retain their textures and flavors.

3. **Consider Cooking Times:** Take into account the cooking times of different ingredients when layering them in the slow cooker. Place ingredients that require longer cooking times, such as root vegetables or tougher cuts of meat, closer to the bottom of the slow cooker where they will be exposed to direct heat and cook more quickly.

4. **Utilize Cooking Times:** Take advantage of the slow cooker's gentle heat by strategically layering ingredients based on their cooking times. Place ingredients that require longer cooking times closer to the heat source, such as root vegetables and tougher cuts of meat. This ensures that these ingredients have sufficient time to tenderize and develop rich flavors during the slow cooking process.

5. **Add Flavor Enhancers:** Enhance the depth of flavor in your slow cooker meals by incorporating flavor enhancers between layers of ingredients. Consider adding aromatics like bay leaves, dried herbs, or spice blends to infuse the dish with complex and aromatic flavors as it cooks. These flavor enhancers gradually release their essence into the surrounding ingredients, resulting in a more flavorful and satisfying meal for your dog.

Avoid Overfilling

1. **Leave Room for Expansion:** Avoid filling the slow cooker more than two-thirds full to allow room for ingredients to expand as they cook. Overfilling the slow cooker can lead to spills or overflow during cooking and may result in unevenly cooked dishes.

2. **Use the Right Size:** Choose a slow cooker that matches the quantity of food you plan to prepare to avoid overfilling. If you're cooking a smaller batch, opt for a smaller slow cooker to ensure optimal cooking results.

3. **Mindful Ingredient Selection:** Practice mindful ingredient selection to prevent overfilling the slow cooker. Choose ingredients that will cook down or soften during the cooking process, allowing ample space for expansion without overcrowding the appliance. Opt for smaller cuts of meat, diced vegetables, and grains that absorb liquid and expand gently, ensuring that your slow cooker remains within its capacity.

4. **Batch Cooking:** Consider batch cooking larger quantities of dog food and storing portions in the freezer for future use. By preparing multiple meals at once and portioning them into individual servings, you can increase the efficiency of your slow cooker while reducing the risk of overfilling. Batch cooking also allows you to rotate between different recipes and flavors, providing variety in your dog's diet.

Minimize Opening Lid

1. **Preserve Heat and Moisture:** Resist the urge to open the slow cooker lid frequently during cooking, as this allows valuable heat and moisture to escape. Keeping the lid closed helps maintain a consistent cooking temperature and ensures that ingredients cook evenly and thoroughly.

2. **Plan Ahead:** Use a timer or set a cooking schedule to minimize the need to check on the progress of your dog's meals frequently. Trust the slow cooker to do its job and resist the temptation to peek inside until the cooking time is complete.

3. **Transparent Lid:** Invest in a slow cooker with a transparent lid to monitor the cooking progress without lifting the lid. A transparent lid allows you to observe the contents of the slow cooker without disrupting the cooking process, enabling you to assess the texture, color, and aroma of the food as it cooks. This reduces the need to open the lid unnecessarily, preserving heat and moisture within the appliance.

4. **Optimize Cooking Time:** Plan your slow cooker meals to align with your schedule and minimize the temptation to open the lid prematurely. Select recipes with appropriate cooking times that allow for uninterrupted cooking without the need for frequent checks or adjustments. Utilize programmable slow cookers with built-in timers to automatically switch to the "warm" setting once the cooking cycle is complete, ensuring that your dog's meals remain warm and ready to serve until mealtime.

Adjust Seasoning

1. **Choose Dog-Safe Seasonings:** When seasoning your dog's meals, opt for dog-safe herbs and spices that enhance flavor without adding harmful ingredients. Parsley, basil, oregano, and turmeric are excellent choices that add flavor and aroma to your dog's meals without the risk of toxicity.

2. **Experiment with Flavors:** Get creative with seasonings and experiment with different combinations to create delicious and nutritious meals for your dog. Consider incorporating fresh herbs, spices, or natural flavorings like curry powder (in moderation) to add variety to your dog's diet.

3. **Homemade Seasoning Blends:** Create your homemade seasoning blends using dog-friendly ingredients to customize the flavor profile of your dog's meals. Experiment with combinations of dried herbs, spices, and natural flavorings to tailor the seasoning to your dog's preferences and dietary needs. Homemade seasoning blends allow you to control the ingredients and avoid additives or preservatives commonly found in commercial seasoning mixes, ensuring that your dog's meals are wholesome and nutritious.

4. **Taste Test:** Conduct a taste test of your dog's meals before serving to ensure that the seasoning is balanced and palatable. Offer a small sample to your dog and observe their reaction to the flavor and aroma of the dish. Adjust the seasoning as needed based on your dog's preferences and feedback, adding additional herbs or spices to enhance the flavor without overwhelming the dish. Remember to avoid adding salt or salty seasonings, as excessive sodium intake can be harmful to your dog's health.

By choosing the right slow cooker, preparing ingredients properly, and following tips for successful slow cooking, you can create nutritious and delicious meals for your dog with ease. In the following chapters, we'll explore a variety of nutritious recipes for every meal, including meat-based, chicken-based, turkey-based, and fish-based options, created to meet your dog's specific dietary needs and preferences.

Chapter 3

50 NUTRITIOUS RECIPES FOR EVERY MEAL

15

Meat-Based Recipes

Savory Beef Stew

PREP TIME:	COOKING TIME:	SERVINGS:
15 mins	6-8 hours	4-6

INGREDIENTS:

- 1 lb beef stew meat, cubed
- 3 carrots, peeled and sliced
- 2 potatoes, peeled and diced
- 2 stalks celery, chopped
- 4 cups beef broth
- 1 tsp dried thyme
- 1 tsp dried rosemary
- Salt and pepper to taste

PORTION SIZES:

For Small Dogs (under 20 pounds):

- Beef stew meat: 50 grams
- Carrots: 15 grams
- Potatoes: 10 grams
- Celery: 10 grams
- Beef broth: 60 ml

For Medium Dogs (20-50 pounds):

- Beef stew meat: 100 grams
- Carrots: 30 grams
- Potatoes: 20 grams
- Celery: 20 grams
- Beef broth: 120 ml

For Large Dogs (over 50 pounds):

- Beef stew meat: 150 grams
- Carrots: 45 grams
- Potatoes: 30 grams
- Celery: 30 grams
- Beef broth: 180 ml

DIRECTIONS:

1. In a skillet over medium heat, brown the beef cubes on all sides. Transfer to the slow cooker.
2. Add the carrots, potatoes, celery, and beef broth to the slow cooker.
3. Sprinkle the dried thyme and rosemary over the mixture. Season with salt and pepper to taste.
4. Cover and cook on low for 6-8 hours or until the beef is tender.

Nutritional Facts: (per serving, assuming 6 servings)

Calories: 250; Fat: 10g; Carbohydrates: 15g; Protein: 25g; Cholesterol: 75mg; Sodium: 700mg; Potassium: 650mg

Tender Beef and Vegetable Stew

PREP TIME:	COOKING TIME:	SERVINGS:
20 mins	6-8 hours	4-6

INGREDIENTS:

- 1 lb beef chuck roast, cubed
- 2 carrots, peeled and sliced
- 2 stalks celery, chopped
- 2 potatoes, peeled and diced
- 4 cups beef broth
- 1 can diced tomatoes, undrained
- 1 cup frozen peas
- 1 tsp dried thyme
- Salt and pepper to taste

PORTION SIZES:

For Small Dogs (under 20 pounds):

- Beef chuck roast: 50 grams
- Carrots: 15 grams
- Celery: 15 grams
- Potatoes: 15 grams
- Beef broth: 60 ml
- Diced tomatoes: 15 grams
- Frozen peas: 10 grams

For Medium Dogs (20-50 pounds):

- Beef chuck roast: 100 grams
- Carrots: 30 grams
- Celery: 30 grams
- Potatoes: 30 grams
- Beef broth: 120 ml
- Diced tomatoes: 30 grams
- Frozen peas: 20 grams

For Large Dogs (over 50 pounds):

- Beef chuck roast: 150 grams
- Carrots: 45 grams
- Celery: 45 grams
- Potatoes: 45 grams
- Beef broth: 180 ml
- Diced tomatoes: 45 grams
- Frozen peas: 30 grams

DIRECTIONS:

1. Brown the beef cubes in a skillet over medium heat. Transfer to the slow cooker.
2. Add the carrots, celery, potatoes, diced tomatoes, and frozen peas to the slow cooker.
3. Pour the beef broth over the ingredients in the slow cooker.
4. Sprinkle the dried thyme over the mixture. Season with salt and pepper to taste.
5. Cover and cook on low for 6-8 hours or until the beef is tender.

Nutritional Facts: (per serving, assuming 6 servings)

Calories: 280; Fat: 12g; Carbohydrates: 15g; Protein: 28g; Cholesterol: 80mg; Sodium: 750mg; Potassium: 680mg

Classic Beef and Potato Stew

PREP TIME:	COOKING TIME:	SERVINGS:
15 mins	6-8 hours	4-6

INGREDIENTS:

- 1 lb beef stew meat, cubed
- 3 potatoes, peeled and diced
- 2 carrots, peeled and sliced
- 2 stalks celery, chopped
- 4 cups beef broth
- 1 cup frozen corn kernels
- 1 tsp dried thyme
- Salt and pepper to taste

PORTION SIZES:

For Small Dogs (under 20 pounds):

- Beef stew meat: 50 grams
- Potatoes: 20 grams
- Carrots: 15 grams
- Celery: 15 grams
- Beef broth: 60 ml
- Frozen corn kernels: 10 grams

For Medium Dogs (20-50 pounds):

- Beef stew meat: 100 grams
- Potatoes: 40 grams
- Carrots: 30 grams
- Celery: 30 grams
- Beef broth: 120 ml
- Frozen corn kernels: 20 grams

For Large Dogs (over 50 pounds):

- Beef stew meat: 150 grams
- Potatoes: 60 grams
- Carrots: 45 grams
- Celery: 45 grams
- Beef broth: 180 ml
- Frozen corn kernels: 30 grams

DIRECTIONS:

1. Brown the beef cubes in a skillet over medium heat. Transfer to the slow cooker.
2. Add the potatoes, carrots, celery, frozen corn kernels, and beef broth to the slow cooker.
3. Sprinkle the dried thyme over the mixture. Season with salt and pepper to taste.
4. Cover and cook on low for 6-8 hours or until the beef is tender.

Nutritional Facts: (per serving, assuming 6 servings)

Calories: 270; Fat: 10g; Carbohydrates: 20g; Protein: 25g; Cholesterol: 70mg; Sodium: 800mg; Potassium: 600mg

Hearty Beef and Barley Stew

PREP TIME:	**COOKING TIME:**	**SERVINGS:**
20 mins	6-8 hours	4-6

INGREDIENTS:

- 1 lb beef stew meat, cubed
- 1 cup pearl barley
- 3 carrots, peeled and sliced
- 2 stalks celery, chopped
- 1 can diced tomatoes, undrained
- 4 cups beef broth
- 1 tsp dried thyme
- Salt and pepper to taste

PORTION SIZES:

For Small Dogs (under 20 pounds):

- Beef stew meat: 50 grams
- Pearl barley: 10 grams
- Carrots: 15 grams
- Celery: 10 grams
- Diced tomatoes: 10 grams
- Beef broth: 60 ml

For Medium Dogs (20-50 pounds):

- Beef stew meat: 100 grams
- Pearl barley: 20 grams
- Carrots: 30 grams
- Celery: 20 grams
- Diced tomatoes: 20 grams
- Beef broth: 120 ml

For Large Dogs (over 50 pounds):

- Beef stew meat: 150 grams
- Pearl barley: 30 grams
- Carrots: 45 grams
- Celery: 30 grams
- Diced tomatoes: 30 grams
- Beef broth: 180 ml

DIRECTIONS:

1. Brown the beef cubes in a skillet over medium heat. Transfer to the slow cooker.
2. Add the pearl barley, carrots, celery, diced tomatoes, and beef broth to the slow cooker.
3. Sprinkle the dried thyme over the mixture. Season with salt and pepper to taste.
4. Cover and cook on low for 6-8 hours or until the beef is tender and the barley is cooked through.

Nutritional Facts: (per serving, assuming 6 servings)

Calories: 320; Fat: 10g; Carbohydrates: 35g; Protein: 25g; Cholesterol: 75mg; Sodium: 750mg; Potassium: 700mg

Beef and Rice Casserole

PREP TIME:	COOKING TIME:	SERVINGS:
20 mins	4-6 hours	4-6

INGREDIENTS:

- 1 lb ground beef
- 1 cup uncooked white rice
- 2 carrots, peeled and diced
- 1 bell pepper, diced
- 1 can diced tomatoes, undrained
- 2 cups beef broth
- 1 tsp dried oregano
- Salt and pepper to taste

PORTION SIZES:

For Small Dogs (under 20 pounds):

- Ground beef: 50 grams
- Uncooked white rice: 10 grams
- Carrots: 10 grams
- Bell pepper: 5 grams
- Diced tomatoes: 5 grams
- Beef broth: 60 ml

For Medium Dogs (20-50 pounds):

- Ground beef: 100 grams
- Uncooked white rice: 20 grams
- Carrots: 20 grams
- Bell pepper: 10 grams
- Diced tomatoes: 10 grams
- Beef broth: 120 ml

For Large Dogs (over 50 pounds):

- Ground beef: 150 grams
- Uncooked white rice: 30 grams
- Carrots: 30 grams
- Bell pepper: 15 grams
- Diced tomatoes: 15 grams
- Beef broth: 180 ml

DIRECTIONS:

1. In a skillet over medium heat, cook the ground beef until browned. Drain excess fat and transfer to the slow cooker.
2. Add the uncooked white rice, diced carrots, diced bell pepper, diced tomatoes, beef broth, dried oregano, salt, and pepper to the slow cooker.
3. Stir to combine all ingredients.
4. Cover and cook on low for 4-6 hours or until the rice is cooked through.

Nutritional Facts: (per serving, assuming 6 servings)

Calories: 320; Fat: 10g; Carbohydrates: 30g; Protein: 25g; Cholesterol: 70mg; Sodium: 750mg; Potassium: 600mg

Beef and Sweet Potato Stew

PREP TIME:	COOKING TIME:	SERVINGS:
20 mins	6-8 hours	4-6

INGREDIENTS:

- 1 lb beef stew meat, cubed
- 2 sweet potatoes, peeled and diced
- 2 carrots, peeled and sliced
- 1 can diced tomatoes, not drained
- 4 cups beef broth
- 1 tsp dried thyme
- Salt and pepper to taste

PORTION SIZES:

For Small Dogs (under 20 pounds):

- Beef stew meat: 50 grams
- Sweet potatoes: 20 grams
- Carrots: 15 grams
- Diced tomatoes: 5 grams
- Beef broth: 60 ml

For Medium Dogs (20-50 pounds):

- Beef stew meat: 100 grams
- Sweet potatoes: 40 grams
- Carrots: 30 grams
- Diced tomatoes: 10 grams
- Beef broth: 120 ml

For Large Dogs (over 50 pounds):

- Beef stew meat: 150 grams
- Sweet potatoes: 60 grams
- Carrots: 45 grams
- Diced tomatoes: 15 grams
- Beef broth: 180 ml

DIRECTIONS:

1. Brown the beef cubes in a skillet over medium heat. Transfer to the slow cooker.
2. Add the diced sweet potatoes, carrots, diced tomatoes, and beef broth to the slow cooker.
3. Sprinkle the dried thyme over the mixture. Season with salt and pepper to taste.
4. Cover and cook on low for 6-8 hours or until the beef is tender and the sweet potatoes are cooked through.

Nutritional Facts: (per serving, assuming 6 servings)

Calories: 300; Fat: 10g; Carbohydrates: 25g; Protein: 25g; Cholesterol: 75mg; Sodium: 750mg; Potassium: 700mg

Beef and Pumpkin Stew

PREP TIME:	COOKING TIME:	SERVINGS:
20 mins	6-8 hours	4-6

INGREDIENTS:

- 1 lb beef stew meat, cubed
- 1 can pumpkin puree
- 2 potatoes, peeled and diced
- 2 carrots, peeled and sliced
- 4 cups beef broth
- 1 tsp dried sage
- Salt and pepper to taste

PORTION SIZES:

For Small Dogs (under 20 pounds):

- Beef stew meat: 50 grams
- Pumpkin puree: 20 grams
- Potatoes: 15 grams
- Carrots: 15 grams
- Beef broth: 60 ml

For Medium Dogs (20-50 pounds):

- Beef stew meat: 100 grams
- Pumpkin puree: 40 grams
- Potatoes: 30 grams
- Carrots: 30 grams
- Beef broth: 120 ml

For Large Dogs (over 50 pounds):

- Beef stew meat: 150 grams
- Pumpkin puree: 60 grams
- Potatoes: 45 grams
- Carrots: 45 grams
- Beef broth: 180 ml

DIRECTIONS:

1. Brown the beef cubes in a skillet over medium heat. Transfer to the slow cooker.
2. Add the pumpkin puree, diced potatoes, carrots, and beef broth to the slow cooker.
3. Sprinkle the dried sage over the mixture. Season with salt and pepper to taste.
4. Cover and cook on low for 6-8 hours or until the beef is tender and the vegetables are cooked through.

Nutritional Facts: (per serving, assuming 6 servings)

Calories: 280; Fat: 10g; Carbohydrates: 20g; Protein: 25g; Cholesterol: 75mg; Sodium: 750mg; Potassium: 700mg

Beef and Green Bean Stew

PREP TIME:	**COOKING TIME:**	**SERVINGS:**
20 mins	6-8 hours	4-6

INGREDIENTS:

- 1 lb beef stew meat, cubed
- 2 cups green beans, trimmed and cut into bite-sized pieces
- 2 potatoes, peeled and diced
- 4 cups beef broth
- 1 tsp dried parsley
- Salt and pepper to taste

PORTION SIZES:

For Small Dogs (under 20 pounds):

- Beef stew meat: 50 grams
- Green beans: 10 grams
- Potatoes: 10 grams
- Beef broth: 60 ml

For Medium Dogs (20-50 pounds):

- Beef stew meat: 100 grams
- Green beans: 20 grams
- Potatoes: 20 grams
- Beef broth: 120 ml

For Large Dogs (over 50 pounds):

- Beef stew meat: 150 grams
- Green beans: 30 grams
- Potatoes: 30 grams
- Beef broth: 180 ml

DIRECTIONS:

1. Brown the beef cubes in a skillet over medium heat. Transfer to the slow cooker.
2. Add the green beans, diced potatoes, and beef broth to the slow cooker.
3. Sprinkle the dried parsley over the mixture. Season with salt and pepper to taste.
4. Cover and cook on low for 6-8 hours or until the beef is tender and the vegetables are cooked through.

Nutritional Facts: (per serving, assuming 6 servings)

Calories: 290; Fat: 10g; Carbohydrates: 25g; Protein: 25g; Cholesterol: 75mg; Sodium: 750mg; Potassium: 700mg

Beef and Butternut Squash Stew

PREP TIME:	COOKING TIME:	SERVINGS:
20 mins	6-8 hours	4-6

INGREDIENTS:

- 1 lb beef stew meat, cubed
- 1 butternut squash, peeled, seeded, and diced
- 2 carrots, peeled and sliced
- 4 cups beef broth
- 1 tsp dried thyme
- Salt and pepper to taste

PORTION SIZES:

For Small Dogs (under 20 pounds):

- Beef stew meat: 50 grams
- Butternut squash: 20 grams
- Carrots: 15 grams
- Beef broth: 60 ml

For Medium Dogs (20-50 pounds):

- Beef stew meat: 100 grams
- Butternut squash: 40 grams
- Carrots: 30 grams
- Beef broth: 120 ml

For Large Dogs (over 50 pounds):

- Beef stew meat: 150 grams
- Butternut squash: 60 grams
- Carrots: 45 grams
- Beef broth: 180 ml

DIRECTIONS:

1. Brown the beef cubes in a skillet over medium heat. Transfer to the slow cooker.
2. Add the diced butternut squash, carrots, and beef broth to the slow cooker.
3. Sprinkle the dried thyme over the mixture. Season with salt and pepper to taste.
4. Cover and cook on low for 6-8 hours or until the beef is tender and the vegetables are cooked through.

Nutritional Facts: (per serving, assuming 6 servings)

Calories: 280; Fat: 10g; Carbohydrates: 25g; Protein: 25g; Cholesterol: 75mg; Sodium: 750mg; Potassium: 700mg

Beef and Zucchini Stew

PREP TIME:	COOKING TIME:	SERVINGS:
20 mins	6-8 hours	4-6

INGREDIENTS:

- 1 lb beef stew meat, cubed
- 2 zucchini, sliced
- 2 potatoes, peeled and diced
- 4 cups beef broth
- 1 tsp dried basil
- Salt and pepper to taste

PORTION SIZES:

For Small Dogs (under 20 pounds):

- Beef stew meat: 50 grams
- Zucchini: 10 grams
- Potatoes: 10 grams
- Beef broth: 60 ml

For Medium Dogs (20-50 pounds):

- Beef stew meat: 100 grams
- Zucchini: 20 grams
- Potatoes: 20 grams
- Beef broth: 120 ml

For Large Dogs (over 50 pounds):

- Beef stew meat: 150 grams
- Zucchini: 30 grams
- Potatoes: 30 grams
- Beef broth: 180 ml

DIRECTIONS:

1. Brown the beef cubes in a skillet over medium heat. Transfer to the slow cooker.
2. Add the sliced zucchini, diced potatoes, and beef broth to the slow cooker.
3. Sprinkle the dried basil over the mixture. Season with salt and pepper to taste.
4. Cover and cook on low for 6-8 hours or until the beef is tender and the vegetables are cooked through.

Nutritional Facts: (per serving, assuming 6 servings)

Calories: 290; Fat: 10g; Carbohydrates: 25g; Protein: 25g; Cholesterol: 75mg; Sodium: 750mg; Potassium: 700mg

Beef and Pea Stew

PREP TIME:	COOKING TIME:	SERVINGS:
20 mins	6-8 hours	4-6

INGREDIENTS:

- 1 lb beef stew meat, cubed
- 2 cups frozen peas
- 2 carrots, peeled and sliced
- 2 potatoes, peeled and diced
- 4 cups beef broth
- 1 tsp dried rosemary
- Salt and pepper to taste

PORTION SIZES:

For Small Dogs (under 20 pounds):

- Beef stew meat: 50 grams
- Frozen peas: 10 grams
- Carrots: 10 grams
- Potatoes: 10 grams
- Beef broth: 60 ml

For Medium Dogs (20-50 pounds):

- Beef stew meat: 100 grams
- Frozen peas: 20 grams
- Carrots: 20 grams
- Potatoes: 20 grams
- Beef broth: 120 ml

For Large Dogs (over 50 pounds):

- Beef stew meat: 150 grams
- Frozen peas: 30 grams
- Carrots: 30 grams
- Potatoes: 30 grams
- Beef broth: 180 ml

DIRECTIONS:

1. Brown the beef cubes in a skillet over medium heat. Transfer to the slow cooker.
2. Add the frozen peas, sliced carrots, diced potatoes, and beef broth to the slow cooker.
3. Sprinkle the dried rosemary over the mixture. Season with salt and pepper to taste.
4. Cover and cook on low for 6-8 hours or until the beef is tender and the vegetables are cooked through.

Nutritional Facts: (per serving, assuming 6 servings)

Calories: 280; Fat: 10g; Carbohydrates: 25g; Protein: 25g; Cholesterol: 75mg; Sodium: 750mg; Potassium: 700mg

Beef and Carrot Casserole

PREP TIME:	COOKING TIME:	SERVINGS:
20 mins	4-6 hours	4-6

INGREDIENTS:

- 1 lb beef stew meat, cubed
- 3 carrots, peeled and sliced
- 1 cup frozen peas
- 2 potatoes, peeled and diced
- 1 can (14.5 oz) diced tomatoes, undrained
- 1 cup beef broth
- 1 tsp dried thyme
- Salt and pepper to taste

PORTION SIZES:

For Small Dogs (under 20 pounds):

- Beef stew meat: 50 grams
- Carrots: 10 grams
- Frozen peas: 5 grams
- Potatoes: 10 grams
- Diced tomatoes: 5 grams
- Beef broth: 60 ml

For Medium Dogs (20-50 pounds):

- Beef stew meat: 100 grams
- Carrots: 20 grams
- Frozen peas: 10 grams
- Potatoes: 20 grams
- Diced tomatoes: 10 grams
- Beef broth: 120 ml

For Large Dogs (over 50 pounds):

- Beef stew meat: 150 grams
- Carrots: 30 grams
- Frozen peas: 15 grams
- Potatoes: 30 grams
- Diced tomatoes: 15 grams
- Beef broth: 180 ml

DIRECTIONS:

1. Brown the beef cubes in a skillet over medium heat. Transfer to the slow cooker.
2. Add the sliced carrots, frozen peas, diced potatoes, diced tomatoes, and beef broth to the slow cooker.
3. Sprinkle the dried thyme over the mixture. Season with salt and pepper to taste.
4. Cover and cook on low for 4-6 hours or until the beef is tender and the vegetables are cooked through.

Nutritional Facts: (per serving, assuming 6 servings)

Calories: 280; Fat: 10g; Carbohydrates: 25g; Protein: 25g; Cholesterol: 75mg; Sodium: 750mg; Potassium: 700mg

Lamb and Sweet Potato Stew

PREP TIME:	COOKING TIME:	SERVINGS:
20 mins	6-8 hours	4-6

INGREDIENTS:

- 1 lb lamb shoulder, cubed
- 2 sweet potatoes, peeled and diced
- 2 carrots, peeled and sliced
- 1 can diced tomatoes, undrained
- 4 cups chicken broth
- 1 tsp dried sage
- Salt and pepper to taste

PORTION SIZES:

For Small Dogs (under 20 pounds):

- Lamb shoulder: 50 grams
- Sweet potatoes: 20 grams
- Carrots: 15 grams
- Diced tomatoes: 5 grams
- Chicken broth: 60 ml

For Medium Dogs (20-50 pounds):

- Lamb shoulder: 100 grams
- Sweet potatoes: 40 grams
- Carrots: 30 grams
- Diced tomatoes: 10 grams
- Chicken broth: 120 ml

For Large Dogs (over 50 pounds):

- Lamb shoulder: 150 grams
- Sweet potatoes: 60 grams
- Carrots: 45 grams
- Diced tomatoes: 15 grams
- Chicken broth: 180 ml

DIRECTIONS:

1. Brown the lamb cubes in a skillet over medium heat. Transfer to the slow cooker.
2. Add the diced sweet potatoes, sliced carrots, diced tomatoes, and chicken broth to the slow cooker.
3. Sprinkle the dried sage over the mixture. Season with salt and pepper to taste.
4. Cover and cook on low for 6-8 hours or until the lamb is tender and the vegetables are cooked through.

Nutritional Facts: (per serving, assuming 6 servings)

Calories: 300; Fat: 10g; Carbohydrates: 25g; Protein: 25g; Cholesterol: 75mg; Sodium: 750mg; Potassium: 700mg

Lamb and Lentil Stew

PREP TIME:	**COOKING TIME:**	**SERVINGS:**
20 mins	6-8 hours	4-6

INGREDIENTS:

- 1 lb lamb stew meat, cubed
- 1 cup dried green lentils, rinsed
- 3 carrots, peeled and sliced
- 2 potatoes, peeled and diced
- 4 cups beef broth
- 1 tsp dried rosemary
- Salt and pepper to taste

PORTION SIZES:

For Small Dogs (under 20 pounds):

- Lamb stew meat: 50 grams
- Dried green lentils: 10 grams
- Carrots: 10 grams
- Potatoes: 10 grams
- Beef broth: 60 ml

For Medium Dogs (20-50 pounds):

- Lamb stew meat: 100 grams
- Dried green lentils: 20 grams
- Carrots: 20 grams
- Potatoes: 20 grams
- Beef broth: 120 ml

For Large Dogs (over 50 pounds):

- Lamb stew meat: 150 grams
- Dried green lentils: 30 grams
- Carrots: 30 grams
- Potatoes: 30 grams
- Beef broth: 180 ml

DIRECTIONS:

1. Brown the lamb cubes in a skillet over medium heat. Transfer to the slow cooker.
2. Add the dried green lentils, sliced carrots, diced potatoes, and beef broth to the slow cooker.
3. Sprinkle the dried rosemary over the mixture. Season with salt and pepper to taste.
4. Cover and cook on low for 6-8 hours or until the lamb is tender and the lentils are cooked through.

Nutritional Facts: (per serving, assuming 6 servings)

Calories: 320; Fat: 10g; Carbohydrates: 30g; Protein: 25g; Cholesterol: 80mg; Sodium: 700mg; Potassium: 750mg

Beef and Apple Casserole

PREP TIME:	COOKING TIME:	SERVINGS:
20 mins	6-8 hours	4-6

INGREDIENTS:

- 1 lb beef skirt, cubed
- 2 apples, peeled, cored, and sliced
- 2 sweet potatoes, peeled and diced
- 4 cups chicken broth
- 1 tsp dried thyme
- Salt and pepper to taste

PORTION SIZES:

For Small Dogs (under 20 pounds):

- Beef skirt: 50 grams
- Apples: 20 grams
- Sweet potatoes: 10 grams
- Chicken broth: 60 ml

For Medium Dogs (20-50 pounds):

- Beef skirt: 100 grams
- Apples: 40 grams
- Sweet potatoes: 20 grams
- Chicken broth: 120 ml

For Large Dogs (over 50 pounds):

- Beef skirt: 150 grams
- Apples: 60 grams
- Sweet potatoes: 30 grams
- Chicken broth: 180 ml

DIRECTIONS:

1. Brown the beef cubes in a skillet over medium heat. Transfer to the slow cooker.
2. Add the sliced apples, diced sweet potatoes, chicken broth, dried thyme, salt, and pepper to the slow cooker.
3. Stir to combine all ingredients.
4. Cover and cook on low for 6-8 hours or until the beef is tender and the vegetables are cooked through.

Nutritional Facts: (per serving, assuming 6 servings)

Calories: 280; Fat: 8g; Carbohydrates: 30g; Protein: 25g; Cholesterol: 70mg; Sodium: 750mg; Potassium: 700mg

15

Chicken-Based Recipes

Chicken and Sweet Potato Stew

PREP TIME:	COOKING TIME:	SERVINGS:
20 mins	6-8 hours	4-6

INGREDIENTS:

- 1 lb chicken breasts, cubed
- 2 sweet potatoes, peeled and diced
- 2 carrots, peeled and sliced
- 1 can diced tomatoes, undrained
- 4 cups chicken broth
- 1 tsp dried thyme
- Salt and pepper to taste

PORTION SIZES:

For Small Dogs (under 20 pounds):

- Chicken breasts: 50 grams
- Sweet potatoes: 20 grams
- Carrots: 15 grams
- Chicken broth: 60 ml

For Medium Dogs (20-50 pounds):

- Chicken breasts: 100 grams
- Sweet potatoes: 40 grams
- Carrots: 30 grams
- Chicken broth: 120 ml

For Large Dogs (over 50 pounds):

- Chicken breasts: 150 grams
- Sweet potatoes: 60 grams
- Carrots: 45 grams
- Chicken broth: 180 ml

DIRECTIONS:

1. Place the cubed chicken breasts in the slow cooker.
2. Add the diced sweet potatoes, sliced carrots, diced tomatoes, chicken broth, dried thyme, salt, and pepper to the slow cooker.
3. Stir to combine all ingredients.
4. Cover and cook on low for 6-8 hours or until the chicken is cooked through and the vegetables are tender.

Nutritional Facts: (per serving, assuming 6 servings)

Calories: 250; Fat: 4g; Carbohydrates: 25g; Protein: 30g; Cholesterol: 75mg; Sodium: 700mg; Potassium: 750mg

Chicken and Butternut Squash Stew

PREP TIME:	COOKING TIME:	SERVINGS:
20 mins	6-8 hours	4-6

INGREDIENTS:

- 1 lb chicken thighs, boneless and skinless, cubed
- 1 butternut squash, peeled, seeded, and diced
- 2 carrots, peeled and sliced
- 1 can diced tomatoes, undrained
- 4 cups chicken broth
- 1 tsp dried sage
- Salt and pepper to taste

PORTION SIZES:

For Small Dogs (under 20 pounds):

- Chicken thighs: 50 grams
- Butternut squash: 20 grams
- Carrots: 15 grams
- Chicken broth: 60 ml

For Medium Dogs (20-50 pounds):

- Chicken thighs: 100 grams
- Butternut squash: 40 grams
- Carrots: 30 grams
- Chicken broth: 120 ml

For Large Dogs (over 50 pounds):

- Chicken thighs: 150 grams
- Butternut squash: 60 grams
- Carrots: 45 grams
- Chicken broth: 180 ml

DIRECTIONS:

1. Place the cubed chicken thighs in the slow cooker.
2. Add the diced butternut squash, sliced carrots, diced tomatoes, chicken broth, dried sage, salt, and pepper to the slow cooker.
3. Stir to combine all ingredients.
4. Cover and cook on low for 6-8 hours or until the chicken is cooked through and the squash is tender.

Nutritional Facts: (per serving, assuming 6 servings)

Calories: 280; Fat: 6g; Carbohydrates: 30g; Protein: 28g; Cholesterol: 80mg; Sodium: 750mg; Potassium: 700mg

Chicken and Pea Casserole

PREP TIME:	COOKING TIME:	SERVINGS:
20 mins	6-8 hours	4-6

INGREDIENTS:

- 1 lb chicken thighs, boneless and skinless, cubed
- 2 cups frozen peas
- 2 carrots, peeled and sliced
- 2 potatoes, peeled and diced
- 4 cups chicken broth
- 1 tsp dried parsley
- Salt and pepper to taste

PORTION SIZES:

For Small Dogs (under 20 pounds):

- Chicken thighs: 50 grams
- Frozen peas: 10 grams
- Carrots: 10 grams
- Potatoes: 10 grams
- Chicken broth: 60 ml

For Medium Dogs (20-50 pounds):

- Chicken thighs: 100 grams
- Frozen peas: 20 grams
- Carrots: 20 grams
- Potatoes: 20 grams
- Chicken broth: 120 ml

For Large Dogs (over 50 pounds):

- Chicken thighs: 150 grams
- Frozen peas: 30 grams
- Carrots: 30 grams
- Potatoes: 30 grams
- Chicken broth: 180 ml

DIRECTIONS:

1. Place the cubed chicken thighs in the slow cooker.
2. Add the frozen peas, sliced carrots, diced potatoes, chicken broth, dried parsley, salt, and pepper to the slow cooker.
3. Stir to combine all ingredients.
4. Cover and cook on low for 6-8 hours or until the chicken is cooked through and the vegetables are tender.

Nutritional Facts: (per serving, assuming 6 servings)

Calories: 270; Fat: 6g; Carbohydrates: 25g; Protein: 28g; Cholesterol: 80mg; Sodium: 750mg; Potassium: 700mg

Chicken and Pumpkin Stew

PREP TIME:	COOKING TIME:	SERVINGS:
20 mins	6-8 hours	4-6

INGREDIENTS:

- 1 lb chicken breasts, cubed
- 1 can pumpkin puree
- 2 carrots, peeled and sliced
- 2 potatoes, peeled and diced
- 4 cups chicken broth
- 1 tsp dried thyme
- Salt and pepper to taste

PORTION SIZES:

For Small Dogs (under 20 pounds):

- Chicken breasts: 50 grams
- Pumpkin puree: 20 grams
- Carrots: 15 grams
- Potatoes: 15 grams
- Chicken broth: 60 ml

For Medium Dogs (20-50 pounds):

- Chicken breasts: 100 grams
- Pumpkin puree: 40 grams
- Carrots: 30 grams
- Potatoes: 30 grams
- Chicken broth: 120 ml

For Large Dogs (over 50 pounds):

- Chicken breasts: 150 grams
- Pumpkin puree: 60 grams
- Carrots: 45 grams
- Potatoes: 45 grams
- Chicken broth: 180 ml

DIRECTIONS:

1. Place the cubed chicken breasts in the slow cooker.
2. Add the pumpkin puree, sliced carrots, diced potatoes, chicken broth, dried thyme, salt, and pepper to the slow cooker.
3. Stir to combine all ingredients.
4. Cover and cook on low for 6-8 hours or until the chicken is cooked through and the vegetables are tender.

Nutritional Facts: (per serving, assuming 6 servings)

Calories: 260; Fat: 3g; Carbohydrates: 30g; Protein: 30g; Cholesterol: 75mg; Sodium: 700mg; Potassium: 750mg

Chicken and Carrot Casserole

PREP TIME:	COOKING TIME:	SERVINGS:
20 mins	6-8 hours	4-6

INGREDIENTS:

- 1 lb chicken thighs, boneless and skinless, cubed
- 3 carrots, peeled and sliced
- 1 cup frozen peas
- 2 potatoes, peeled and diced
- 4 cups chicken broth
- 1 tsp dried rosemary
- Salt and pepper to taste

PORTION SIZES:

For Small Dogs (under 20 pounds):

- Chicken thighs: 50 grams
- Carrots: 15 grams
- Frozen peas: 5 grams
- Potatoes: 15 grams
- Chicken broth: 60 ml

For Medium Dogs (20-50 pounds):

- Chicken thighs: 100 grams
- Carrots: 30 grams
- Frozen peas: 10 grams
- Potatoes: 30 grams
- Chicken broth: 120 ml

For Large Dogs (over 50 pounds):

- Chicken thighs: 150 grams
- Carrots: 45 grams
- Frozen peas: 15 grams
- Potatoes: 45 grams
- Chicken broth: 180 ml

DIRECTIONS:

1. Place the cubed chicken thighs in the slow cooker.
2. Add the sliced carrots, frozen peas, diced potatoes, chicken broth, dried rosemary, salt, and pepper to the slow cooker.
3. Stir to combine all ingredients.
4. Cover and cook on low for 6-8 hours or until the chicken is cooked through and the vegetables are tender.

Nutritional Facts: (per serving, assuming 6 servings)

Calories: 270; Fat: 5g; Carbohydrates: 25g; Protein: 28g; Cholesterol: 80mg; Sodium: 750mg; Potassium: 700mg

Chicken and Green Bean Stew

PREP TIME:	COOKING TIME:	SERVINGS:
20 mins	6-8 hours	4-6

INGREDIENTS:

- 1 lb chicken breasts, cubed
- 2 cups green beans, trimmed and cut into bite-sized pieces
- 2 carrots, peeled and sliced
- 1 can diced tomatoes, undrained
- 4 cups chicken broth
- 1 tsp dried parsley
- Salt and pepper to taste

PORTION SIZES:

For Small Dogs (under 20 pounds):

- Chicken breasts: 50 grams
- Green beans: 10 grams
- Carrots: 15 grams
- Chicken broth: 60 ml

For Medium Dogs (20-50 pounds):

- Chicken breasts: 100 grams
- Green beans: 20 grams
- Carrots: 30 grams
- Chicken broth: 120 ml

For Large Dogs (over 50 pounds):

- Chicken breasts: 150 grams
- Green beans: 30 grams
- Carrots: 45 grams
- Chicken broth: 180 ml

DIRECTIONS:

1. Place the cubed chicken breasts in the slow cooker.
2. Add the green beans, sliced carrots, diced tomatoes, chicken broth, dried parsley, salt, and pepper to the slow cooker.
3. Stir to combine all ingredients.
4. Cover and cook on low for 6-8 hours or until the chicken is cooked through and the vegetables are tender.

Nutritional Facts: (per serving, assuming 6 servings)

Calories: 250; Fat: 3g; Carbohydrates: 25g; Protein: 30g; Cholesterol: 75mg; Sodium: 700mg; Potassium: 750mg

Chicken and Spinach Stew

PREP TIME:	COOKING TIME:	SERVINGS:
20 mins	6-8 hours	4-6

INGREDIENTS:

- 1 lb chicken breasts, cubed
- 4 cups fresh spinach leaves
- 2 carrots, peeled and sliced
- 1 can diced tomatoes, undrained
- 4 cups chicken broth
- 1 tsp dried basil
- Salt and pepper to taste

PORTION SIZES:

For Small Dogs (under 20 pounds):

- Chicken breasts: 50 grams
- Fresh spinach leaves: 10 grams
- Carrots: 15 grams
- Chicken broth: 60 ml

For Medium Dogs (20-50 pounds):

- Chicken breasts: 100 grams
- Fresh spinach leaves: 20 grams
- Carrots: 30 grams
- Chicken broth: 120 ml

For Large Dogs (over 50 pounds):

- Chicken breasts: 150 grams
- Fresh spinach leaves: 30 grams
- Carrots: 45 grams
- Chicken broth: 180 ml

DIRECTIONS:

1. Place the cubed chicken breasts in the slow cooker.
2. Add the fresh spinach leaves, sliced carrots, diced tomatoes, chicken broth, dried basil, salt, and pepper to the slow cooker.
3. Stir to combine all ingredients.
4. Cover and cook on low for 6-8 hours or until the chicken is cooked through and the spinach is wilted.

Nutritional Facts: (per serving, assuming 6 servings)

Calories: 260; Fat: 3g; Carbohydrates: 25g; Protein: 30g; Cholesterol: 75mg; Sodium: 700mg; Potassium: 750mg

Chicken and Broccoli Casserole

PREP TIME:	COOKING TIME:	SERVINGS:
20 mins	6-8 hours	4-6

INGREDIENTS:

- 1 lb chicken thighs, boneless and skinless, cubed
- 2 cups broccoli florets
- 2 carrots, peeled and sliced
- 1 can cream of chicken soup
- 4 cups chicken broth
- 1 tsp dried thyme
- Salt and pepper to taste

PORTION SIZES:

For Small Dogs (under 20 pounds):

- Chicken breasts: 50 grams
- Broccoli florets: 10 grams
- Carrots: 15 grams
- Chicken broth: 60 ml

For Medium Dogs (20-50 pounds):

- Chicken thighs: 100 grams
- Broccoli florets: 20 grams
- Carrots: 30 grams
- Chicken broth: 120 ml

For Large Dogs (over 50 pounds):

- Chicken thighs: 150 grams
- Broccoli florets: 30 grams
- Carrots: 45 grams
- Chicken broth: 180 ml

DIRECTIONS:

1. Place the cubed chicken thighs in the slow cooker.
2. Add the broccoli florets, sliced carrots, cream of chicken soup, chicken broth, dried thyme, salt, and pepper to the slow cooker.
3. Stir to combine all ingredients.
4. Cover and cook on low for 6-8 hours or until the chicken is cooked through and the broccoli is tender.

Nutritional Facts: (per serving, assuming 6 servings)

Calories: 280; Fat: 6g; Carbohydrates: 25g; Protein: 28g; Cholesterol: 80mg; Sodium: 750mg; Potassium: 700mg

Chicken and Carrot Soup

PREP TIME:	COOKING TIME:	SERVINGS:
15 mins	6-8 hours	4-6

INGREDIENTS:

- 1 lb chicken breasts, cubed
- 3 carrots, peeled and sliced
- 1 cup celery, sliced
- 4 cups chicken broth
- 1 tsp dried parsley
- Salt and pepper to taste

PORTION SIZES:

For Small Dogs (under 20 pounds):

- Chicken breasts: 50 grams
- Celery: 10 grams
- Carrots: 15 grams
- Chicken broth: 60 ml

For Medium Dogs (20-50 pounds):

- Chicken breasts: 100 grams
- Celery: 20 grams
- Carrots: 30 grams
- Chicken broth: 120 ml

For Large Dogs (over 50 pounds):

- Chicken breasts: 150 grams
- Celery: 30 grams
- Carrots: 45 grams
- Chicken broth: 180 ml

DIRECTIONS:

1. Place the cubed chicken breasts, sliced carrots, and celery in the slow cooker.
2. Add the chicken broth, dried parsley, salt, and pepper to the slow cooker.
3. Stir to combine all ingredients.
4. Cover and cook on low for 6-8 hours or until the chicken is cooked through and the vegetables are tender.

Nutritional Facts: (per serving, assuming 6 servings)

Calories: 200; Fat: 3g; Carbohydrates: 10g; Protein: 30g; Cholesterol: 75mg; Sodium: 700mg; Potassium: 550mg

Chicken and Green Pepper Casserole

PREP TIME:	COOKING TIME:	SERVINGS:
20 mins	6-8 hours	4-6

INGREDIENTS:

- 1 lb chicken thighs, boneless and skinless, cubed
- 2 green bell peppers, diced
- 1 cup corn kernels (fresh or frozen)
- 1 can diced tomatoes, undrained
- 4 cups chicken broth
- 1 tsp dried oregano
- Salt and pepper to taste

PORTION SIZES:

For Small Dogs (under 20 pounds):

- Chicken thighs: 50 grams
- Green bell peppers: 10 grams
- Corn kernel: 5 grams
- Chicken broth: 60 ml

For Medium Dogs (20-50 pounds):

- Chicken thighs: 100 grams
- Green bell peppers: 20 grams
- Corn kernel: 10 grams
- Chicken broth: 120 ml

For Large Dogs (over 50 pounds):

- Chicken thighs: 150 grams
- Green bell peppers: 30 grams
- Corn kernel: 15 grams
- Chicken broth: 180 ml

DIRECTIONS:

1. Place the cubed chicken thighs, diced green peppers, corn kernels, and diced tomatoes in the slow cooker.
2. Add the chicken broth, dried oregano, salt, and pepper to the slow cooker.
3. Stir to combine all ingredients.
4. Cover and cook on low for 6-8 hours or until the chicken is cooked through and the vegetables are tender.

Nutritional Facts: (per serving, assuming 6 servings)

Calories: 250; Fat: 5g; Carbohydrates: 20g; Protein: 28g; Cholesterol: 80mg; Sodium: 750mg; Potassium: 650mg

Chicken and Mushroom Stew

PREP TIME:	COOKING TIME:	SERVINGS:
20 mins	6-8 hours	4-6

INGREDIENTS:

- 1 lb chicken breasts, cubed
- 2 cups sliced mushrooms
- 4 cups chicken broth
- 1 tsp dried thyme
- Salt and pepper to taste

PORTION SIZES:

For Small Dogs (under 20 pounds):

- Chicken breasts: 50 grams
- Sliced mushrooms: 20 grams
- Chicken broth: 60 ml

For Medium Dogs (20-50 pounds):

- Chicken breasts: 100 grams
- Celery: 40 grams
- Chicken broth: 120 ml

For Large Dogs (over 50 pounds):

- Chicken breasts: 150 grams
- Celery: 60 grams
- Chicken broth: 180 ml

DIRECTIONS:

1. Place the cubed chicken breasts and sliced mushrooms in the slow cooker.
2. Add the chicken broth, dried thyme, salt, and pepper to the slow cooker.
3. Stir to combine all ingredients.
4. Cover and cook on low for 6-8 hours or until the chicken is cooked through and the mushrooms are tender.

Nutritional Facts: (per serving, assuming 6 servings)

Calories: 220; Fat: 3g; Carbohydrates: 10g; Protein: 30g; Cholesterol: 75mg; Sodium: 700mg; Potassium: 600mg

Chicken and Zucchini Soup

PREP TIME:	COOKING TIME:	SERVINGS:
15 mins	6-8 hours	4-6

INGREDIENTS:

- 1 lb chicken thighs, boneless and skinless, cubed
- 2 zucchinis, sliced
- 1 cup chopped spinach
- 4 cups chicken broth
- 1 tsp dried basil
- Salt and pepper to taste

PORTION SIZES:

For Small Dogs (under 20 pounds):

- Chicken thighs: 50 grams
- Zucchini: 10 grams
- Chopped spinach: 5 grams
- Chicken broth: 60 ml

For Medium Dogs (20-50 pounds):

- Chicken thigh: 100 grams
- Zucchini: 20 grams
- Chopped spinach: 10 grams
- Chicken broth: 120 ml

For Large Dogs (over 50 pounds):

- Chicken thigh: 150 grams
- Zucchini: 30 grams
- Chopped: 15 grams
- Chicken broth: 180 ml

DIRECTIONS:

1. Place the cubed chicken thighs, sliced zucchini, and chopped spinach in the slow cooker.
2. Add the chicken broth, dried basil, salt, and pepper to the slow cooker.
3. Stir to combine all ingredients.
4. Cover and cook on low for 6-8 hours or until the chicken is cooked through and the vegetables are tender.

Nutritional Facts: (per serving, assuming 6 servings)

Calories: 240; Fat: 4g; Carbohydrates: 10g; Protein: 30g; Cholesterol: 80mg; Sodium: 750mg; Potassium: 650mg

Chicken and Cauliflower Curry

PREP TIME:	COOKING TIME:	SERVINGS:
20 mins	6-8 hours	4-6

INGREDIENTS:

- 1 lb chicken thighs, boneless and skinless, cubed
- 1 head cauliflower, cut into florets
- 1 can of coconut milk
- 2 tbsp curry powder
- 4 cups chicken broth
- Salt and pepper to taste

PORTION SIZES:

For Small Dogs (under 20 pounds):

- Chicken thighs: 50 grams
- Cauliflower florets: 10 grams
- Coconut milk: 20 ml
- Curry powder: ½ tsp
- Chicken broth: 60 ml

For Medium Dogs (20-50 pounds):

- Chicken thighs: 150 grams
- Cauliflower florets: 20 grams
- Coconut milk: 40 ml
- Curry powder: 1 tsp
- Chicken broth: 120 ml

For Large Dogs (over 50 pounds):

- Chicken thighs: 150 grams
- Cauliflower florets: 30 grams
- Coconut milk: 60 ml
- Curry powder: 1½ tsp
- Chicken broth: 180 ml

DIRECTIONS:

1. Place the cubed chicken thighs and cauliflower florets in the slow cooker.
2. In a bowl, mix the coconut milk, curry powder, chicken broth, salt, and pepper. Pour the mixture over the chicken and cauliflower into the slow cooker.
3. Stir to combine all ingredients.
4. Cover and cook on low for 6-8 hours or until the chicken is cooked through and the cauliflower is tender.

Nutritional Facts: (per serving, assuming 6 servings)

Calories: 290; Fat: 15g; Carbohydrates: 10g; Protein: 30g; Cholesterol: 80mg; Sodium: 750mg; Potassium: 650mg

Chicken and Corn Chowder

PREP TIME:	COOKING TIME:	SERVINGS:
20 mins	6-8 hours	4-6

INGREDIENTS:

- 1 lb chicken thighs, boneless and skinless, cubed
- 2 cups corn kernels (fresh or frozen)
- 2 potatoes, peeled and diced
- 4 cups chicken broth
- 1 cup milk
- Salt and pepper to taste

PORTION SIZES:

For Small Dogs (under 20 pounds):

- Chicken thighs: 50 grams
- Corn kernel: 10 grams
- Potatoes: 20 grams
- Chicken broth: 100 ml
- Milk: 20 ml

For Medium Dogs (20-50 pounds):

- Chicken thighs: 100 grams
- Corn kernel: 20 grams
- Potatoes: 40 grams
- Chicken broth: 200 ml
- Milk: 40 ml

For Large Dogs (over 50 pounds):

- Chicken thighs: 150 grams
- Corn kernel: 30 grams
- Potatoes: 60 grams
- Chicken broth: 300 ml
- Milk: 60 ml

DIRECTIONS:

1. Place the cubed chicken thighs, corn kernels, and diced potatoes, into the slow cooker.
2. Add the chicken broth, milk, salt, and pepper to the slow cooker.
3. Stir to combine all ingredients.
4. Cover and cook on low for 6-8 hours or until the chicken is cooked through and the potatoes are tender.

Nutritional Facts: (per serving, assuming 6 servings)

Calories: 280; Fat: 5g; Carbohydrates: 30g; Protein: 28g; Cholesterol: 80mg; Sodium: 750mg; Potassium: 700mg

Chicken and Tomato Soup

PREP TIME:	COOKING TIME:	SERVINGS:
15 mins	6-8 hours	4-6

INGREDIENTS:

- 1 lb chicken breasts, cubed
- 1 can diced tomatoes, undrained
- 2 carrots, peeled and sliced
- 1 celery stalk, sliced
- 4 cups chicken broth
- 1 tsp dried basil
- Salt and pepper to taste

PORTION SIZES:

For Small Dogs (under 20 pounds):

- Chicken breasts: 50 grams
- Diced tomatoes: 10 grams
- Carrots: 10 grams
- Celery: 5 grams
- Chicken broth: 100 ml

For Medium Dogs (20-50 pounds):

- Chicken breasts: 100 grams
- Diced tomatoes: 20 grams
- Carrots: 20 grams
- Celery: 10 grams
- Chicken broth: 200 ml

For Large Dogs (over 50 pounds):

- Chicken breasts: 150 grams
- Diced tomatoes: 30 grams
- Carrots: 30 grams
- Celery: 20 grams
- Chicken broth: 300 ml

DIRECTIONS:

1. Place the cubed chicken breasts, diced tomatoes, sliced carrots, and sliced celery in the slow cooker.
2. Add the chicken broth, dried basil, salt, and pepper to the slow cooker.
3. Stir to combine all ingredients.
4. Cover and cook on low for 6-8 hours or until the chicken is cooked through and the vegetables are tender.

Nutritional Facts: (per serving, assuming 6 servings)

Calories: 230; Fat: 3g; Carbohydrates: 15g; Protein: 30g; Cholesterol: 75mg; Sodium: 700mg; Potassium: 700mg

10
Turkey-Based Recipes

Turkey and Vegetable Stew

PREP TIME:	COOKING TIME:	SERVINGS:
20 mins	6-8 hours	4-6

INGREDIENTS:

- 1 lb turkey breast, cubed
- 2 carrots, peeled and sliced
- 2 potatoes, peeled and diced
- 1 cup green beans, trimmed and cut into bite-sized pieces
- 4 cups turkey or chicken broth
- 1 tsp dried thyme
- Salt and pepper to taste

PORTION SIZES:

For Small Dogs (under 20 pounds):

- Turkey breasts: 50 grams
- Carrots: 10 grams
- Potatoes: 10 grams
- Green beans: 5 grams
- Turkey broth: 100 ml

For Medium Dogs (20-50 pounds):

- Turkey breasts: 100 grams
- Carrots: 20 grams
- Potatoes: 20 grams
- Green beans: 10 grams
- Turkey broth: 200 ml

For Large Dogs (over 50 pounds):

- Turkey breasts: 150 grams
- Carrots: 30 grams
- Potatoes: 30 grams
- Green beans: 15 grams
- Turkey broth: 300 ml

DIRECTIONS:

1. Place the cubed turkey breast, sliced carrots, diced potatoes, and green beans in the slow cooker.
2. Add the turkey or chicken broth, dried thyme, salt, and pepper to the slow cooker.
3. Stir to combine all ingredients.
4. Cover and cook on low for 6-8 hours or until the turkey is cooked through and the vegetables are tender.

Nutritional Facts: (per serving, assuming 6 servings)

Calories: 250; Fat: 3g; Carbohydrates: 25g; Protein: 30g; Cholesterol: 75mg; Sodium: 700mg; Potassium: 750mg

Turkey and Sweet Potato

PREP TIME:	COOKING TIME:	SERVINGS:
20 mins	6-8 hours	4-6

INGREDIENTS:

- 1 lb ground turkey
- 2 sweet potatoes, peeled and diced
- 1 bell pepper, diced
- 1 can diced tomatoes, undrained
- 1 can black beans, drained and rinsed
- 1 cup chicken broth
- Salt and pepper to taste

PORTION SIZES:

For Small Dogs (under 20 pounds):

- Ground turkey: 50 grams
- Sweet potatoes: 20 grams
- Bell pepper: 10 grams
- Diced tomatoes: 10 grams
- Black beans: 10 grams
- Chicken broth: 30 ml

For Medium Dogs (20-50 pounds):

- Ground turkey: 100 grams
- Sweet potatoes: 40 grams
- Bell pepper: 20 grams
- Diced tomatoes: 20 grams
- Black beans: 20 grams
- Chicken broth: 60 ml

For Large Dogs (over 50 pounds):

- Ground turkey: 150 grams
- Sweet potatoes: 60 grams
- Bell pepper: 30 grams
- Diced tomatoes: 30 grams
- Black beans: 30 grams
- Chicken broth: 90 ml

DIRECTIONS:

1. In a skillet, cook the ground turkey until browned. Drain any excess fat.
2. Transter the cooked turkey to the slow cooker.
3. Add the diced sweet potatoes, diced bell pepper, diced tomatoes, black beans, chicken broth, salt, and pepper to the slow cooker.
4. Stir to combine all ingredients.
5. Cover and cook on low for 6-8 hours or until the sweet potatoes are tender.

Nutritional Facts: (per serving, assuming 6 servings)

Calories: 280; Fat: 5g; Carbohydrates: 30g; Protein: 30g; Cholesterol: 75mg; Sodium: 700mg; Potassium: 750mg

Turkey and Lentil Soup

PREP TIME:	**COOKING TIME:**	**SERVINGS:**
20 mins	6-8 hours	4-6

INGREDIENTS:

- 1 lb ground turkey
- 1 cup dried green lentils, rinsed
- 2 carrots, peeled and sliced
- 1 celery stalk, sliced
- 4 cups chicken broth
- 1 tsp dried thyme
- Salt and pepper to taste

PORTION SIZES:

For Small Dogs (under 20 pounds):

- Ground turkey: 50 grams
- Dried green lentils: 10 grams
- Carrots: 10 grams
- Celery: 5 grams
- Chicken broth: 100 ml

For Medium Dogs (20-50 pounds):

- Ground turkey: 100 grams
- Dried green lentils: 20 grams
- Carrots: 20 grams
- Celery: 10 grams
- Chicken broth: 200 ml

For Large Dogs (over 50 pounds):

- Ground turkey: 150 grams
- Dried green lentils: 30 grams
- Carrots: 30 grams
- Celery: 15 grams
- Chicken broth: 300 ml

DIRECTIONS:

1. In a skillet, cook the ground turkey until browned. Drain any excess fat.
2. Transfer the cooked turkey to the slow cooker.
3. Add the rinsed green lentils, sliced carrots, sliced celery, chicken broth, dried thyme, salt, and pepper to the slow cooker.
4. Stir to combine all ingredients.
5. Cover and cook on low for 6-8 hours or until the lentils are tender.

Nutritional Facts: (per serving, assuming 6 servings)

Calories: 270; Fat: 4g; Carbohydrates: 25g; Protein: 30g; Cholesterol: 75mg; Sodium: 700mg; Potassium: 750mg

Turkey and Butternut Squash Stew

PREP TIME:	COOKING TIME:	SERVINGS:
20 mins	6-8 hours	4-6

INGREDIENTS:

- 1 lb ground turkey
- 1 butternut squash, peeled and diced
- 2 carrots, peeled and sliced
- 4 cups chicken broth
- 1 tsp dried sage
- Salt and pepper to taste

PORTION SIZES:

For Small Dogs (under 20 pounds):

- Ground turkey: 50 grams
- Butternut squash: 20 grams
- Carrots: 10 grams
- Chicken broth: 100 ml

For Medium Dogs (20-50 pounds):

- Ground turkey: 100 grams
- Butternut squash: 40 grams
- Carrots: 20 grams
- Chicken broth: 200 ml

For Large Dogs (over 50 pounds):

- Ground turkey: 150 grams
- Butternut squash: 60 grams
- Carrots: 30 grams
- Chicken broth: 300 ml

DIRECTIONS:

1. In a skillet, cook the ground turkey until browned. Drain any excess fat.
2. Transfer the cooked turkey to the slow cooker.
3. Add the diced butternut squash, sliced carrots, chicken broth, dried sage, salt, and pepper to the slow cooker.
4. Stir to combine all ingredients.
5. Cover and cook on low for 6-8 hours or until the butternut squash is tender.

Nutritional Facts: (per serving, assuming 6 servings)

Calories: 280; Fat: 5g; Carbohydrates: 30g; Protein: 30g; Cholesterol: 75mg; Sodium: 700mg; Potassium: 750mg

Turkey and Mushroom Casserole

PREP TIME:	COOKING TIME:	SERVINGS:
20 mins	6-8 hours	4-6

INGREDIENTS:

- 1 lb ground turkey
- 2 cups sliced mushrooms
- 1 bell pepper, diced
- 1 can cream of mushroom soup
- 1 cup chicken broth
- 1 tsp dried thyme
- Salt and pepper to taste

PORTION SIZES:

For Small Dogs (under 20 pounds):

- Ground turkey: 50 grams
- Sliced mushrooms: 10 grams
- Bell pepper: 10 grams
- Cream of mushroom soup: 20 grams
- Chicken broth: 50 ml

For Medium Dogs (20-50 pounds):

- Ground turkey: 100 grams
- Sliced mushrooms: 20 grams
- Bell pepper: 20 grams
- Cream of mushroom soup: 40 grams
- Chicken broth: 100 ml

For Large Dogs (over 50 pounds):

- Ground turkey: 150 grams
- Sliced mushrooms: 30 grams
- Bell pepper: 30 grams
- Cream of mushroom soup: 60 grams
- Chicken broth: 150 ml

DIRECTIONS:

1. In a skillet, cook the ground turkey until browned. Drain any excess fat.
2. Transfer the cooked turkey to the slow cooker.
3. Add the sliced mushrooms, diced bell pepper, cream of mushroom soup, chicken broth, dried thyme, salt, and pepper to the slow cooker.
4. Stir to combine all ingredients.
5. Cover and cook on low for 6-8 hours or until the mushrooms are tender.

Nutritional Facts: (per serving, assuming 6 servings)

Calories: 290; Fat: 6g; Carbohydrates: 20g; Protein: 30g; Cholesterol: 75mg; Sodium: 750mg; Potassium: 700mg

Turkey and Barley Soup

PREP TIME:	COOKING TIME:	SERVINGS:
20 mins	6-8 hours	4-6

INGREDIENTS:

- 1 lb ground turkey
- 1 cup pearl barley
- 2 carrots, peeled and sliced
- 1 celery stalk, sliced
- 4 cups chicken broth
- 1 tsp dried rosemary
- Salt and pepper to taste

PORTION SIZES:

For Small Dogs (under 20 pounds):

- Ground turkey: 50 grams
- Pearl barley: 10 grams
- Carrots: 10 grams
- Celery: 5 grams
- Chicken broth: 100 ml

For Medium Dogs (20-50 pounds):

- Ground turkey: 100 grams
- Pearl barley: 20 grams
- Carrots: 20 grams
- Celery: 10 grams
- Chicken broth: 200 ml

For Large Dogs (over 50 pounds):

- Ground turkey: 150 grams
- Pearl barley: 30 grams
- Carrots: 30 grams
- Celery: 15 grams
- Chicken broth: 300 ml

DIRECTIONS:

1. In a skillet, cook the ground turkey until browned. Drain any excess fat.
2. Transfer the cooked turkey to the slow cooker.
3. Add the pearl barley, sliced carrots, sliced celery, chicken broth, dried rosemary, salt, and pepper to the slow cooker.
4. Stir to combine all ingredients.
5. Cover and cook on low for 6-8 hours or until the barley is tender.

Nutritional Facts: (per serving, assuming 6 servings)

Calories: 280; Fat: 5g; Carbohydrates: 30g; Protein: 30g; Cholesterol: 75mg; Sodium: 700mg; Potassium: 750mg

Turkey and Vegetable Curry

PREP TIME:	COOKING TIME:	SERVINGS:
20 mins	6-8 hours	4-6

INGREDIENTS:

- 1 lb ground turkey
- 1 cup diced carrots
- 1 cup diced potatoes
- 1 cup diced bell peppers (assorted colors)
- 1 can of coconut milk
- 2 tbsp curry powder
- 4 cups chicken broth
- Salt and pepper to taste

PORTION SIZES:

For Small Dogs (under 20 pounds):

- Ground turkey: 50 grams
- Diced carrots: 20 grams
- Diced potatoes: 20 grams
- Diced bell pepper: 20 grams
- Coconut milk: 20 ml
- Chicken broth: 100 ml

For Medium Dogs (20-50 pounds):

- Ground turkey: 100 grams
- Diced carrots: 40 grams
- Diced potatoes: 40 grams
- Diced bell pepper: 40 grams
- Coconut milk: 40 ml
- Chicken broth: 200 ml

For Large Dogs (over 50 pounds):

- Ground turkey: 150 grams
- Diced carrots: 60 grams
- Diced potatoes: 60 grams
- Diced bell pepper: 60 grams
- Coconut milk: 60 ml
- Chicken broth: 300 ml

DIRECTIONS:

1. In a skillet, cook the ground turkey until browned. Drain any excess fat.
2. Transfer the cooked turkey to the slow cooker.
3. Add the diced carrots, potatoes, bell peppers, coconut milk, curry powder, chicken broth, salt, and pepper to the slow cooker.
4. Stir to combine all ingredients.
5. Cover and cook on low for 6-8 hours or until the vegetables are tender.

Nutritional Facts: (per serving, assuming 6 servings)

Calories: 290; Fat: 12g; Carbohydrates: 20g; Protein: 25g; Cholesterol: 75mg; Sodium: 700mg; Potassium: 750mg

Turkey and Squash Casserole

PREP TIME:	COOKING TIME:	SERVINGS:
20 mins	6-8 hours	4-6

INGREDIENTS:

- 1 lb ground turkey
- 1 butternut squash, peeled and diced
- 1 zucchini, diced
- 1 yellow squash, diced
- 1 can cream of chicken soup
- 1 cup chicken broth
- Salt and pepper to taste

PORTION SIZES:

For Small Dogs (under 20 pounds):

- Ground turkey: 50 grams
- Butternut squash: 20 grams
- Zucchini: 20 grams
- Yellow squash: 20 grams
- Cream of chicken soup: 20 ml
- Chicken broth: 100 ml

For Medium Dogs (20-50 pounds):

- Ground turkey: 100 grams
- Butternut squash: 40 grams
- Zucchini: 40 grams
- Yellow squash: 40 grams
- Cream of chicken soup: 40 ml
- Chicken broth: 200 ml

For Large Dogs (over 50 pounds):

- Ground turkey: 150 grams
- Butternut squash: 60 grams
- Zucchini: 60 grams
- Yellow squash: 60 grams
- Cream of chicken soup: 60 ml
- Chicken broth: 300 ml

DIRECTIONS:

1. In a skillet, cook the ground turkey until browned. Drain any excess fat.
2. Transfer the cooked turkey to the slow cooker.
3. Add the diced butternut squash, diced zucchini, diced yellow squash, cream of chicken soup, chicken broth, salt, and pepper to the slow cooker.
4. Stir to combine all ingredients.
5. Cover and cook on low for 6-8 hours or until the squash is tender.

Nutritional Facts: (per serving, assuming 6 servings)

Calories: 280; Fat: 5g; Carbohydrates: 30g; Protein: 30g; Cholesterol: 75mg; Sodium: 700mg; Potassium: 750mg

Turkey and Spinach Lasagna

PREP TIME:	COOKING TIME:	SERVINGS:
30 mins	4-6 hours	6-8

INGREDIENTS:

- 1 lb ground turkey
- 8 lasagna noodles, uncooked
- 2 cups spinach, chopped
- 2 cups shredded mozzarella cheese
- 1 can diced tomatoes, drained
- 1 jar marinara sauce
- 1 cup chicken broth
- Salt and pepper to taste

PORTION SIZES:

For Small Dogs (under 20 pounds):

- Ground turkey: 50 grams
- Lasagna noodles: 15 grams
- Chopped spinach: 20 grams
- Shredded mozzarella cheese: 20 grams
- Dried tomatoes: 20 grams
- Marinara sauce: 20 ml
- Chicken broth: 20 ml

For Medium Dogs (20-50 pounds):

- Ground turkey: 100 grams
- Lasagna noodles: 30 grams
- Chopped spinach: 40 grams
- Shredded mozzarella cheese: 40 grams
- Dried tomatoes: 40 grams
- Marinara sauce: 40 ml
- Chicken broth: 40 ml

For Large Dogs (over 50 pounds):

- Ground turkey: 150 grams
- Lasagna noodles: 45 grams
- Chopped spinach: 60 grams
- Shredded mozzarella cheese: 60 grams
- Dried tomatoes: 60 grams
- Marinara sauce: 60 ml
- Chicken broth: 60 ml

DIRECTIONS:

1. In a skillet, cook the ground turkey until browned. Drain any excess fat.
2. In a bowl, mix the diced tomatoes, marinara sauce, and chicken broth.
3. Spread a thin layer of the sauce mixture on the bottom of the slow cooker.
4. Layer uncooked lasagna noodles, cooked ground turkey, chopped spinach, shredded mozzarella cheese, and sauce mixture in the slow cooker, repeating until all ingredients are used, ending with a layer of sauce on top.
5. Cover and cook on low for 4-6 hours or until the noodles are cooked through.
6. Let it sit for 10-15 minutes before serving.

Nutritional Facts: (per serving, assuming 8 servings)

Calories: 350; Fat: 15g; Carbohydrates: 25g; Protein: 25g; Cholesterol: 65mg; Sodium: 700mg; Potassium: 450mg

Turkey and Rice Casserole

PREP TIME:	COOKING TIME:	SERVINGS:
20 mins	6-8 hours	4-6

INGREDIENTS:

- 1 lb ground turkey
- 1 cup uncooked rice
- 2 cups mixed vegetables (peas, carrots, corn)
- 1 can cream of mushroom soup
- 1 cup chicken broth
- Salt and pepper to taste

PORTION SIZES:

For Small Dogs (under 20 pounds):

- Ground turkey: 50 grams
- Rice: 15 grams
- Mixed vegetables: 40 grams
- Cream of mushrooms soup: 20 ml
- Chicken broth: 20 ml

For Medium Dogs (20-50 pounds):

- Ground turkey: 100 grams
- Rice: 30 grams
- Mixed vegetables: 80 grams
- Cream of mushrooms soup: 40 ml
- Chicken broth: 40 ml

For Large Dogs (over 50 pounds):

- Ground turkey: 150 grams
- Rice: 45 grams
- Mixed vegetables: 120 grams
- Cream of mushrooms soup: 60 ml
- Chicken broth: 60 ml

DIRECTIONS:

1. In a skillet, cook the ground turkey until browned. Drain any excess fat.
2. Transfer the cooked turkey to the slow cooker.
3. Add the uncooked rice, mixed vegetables, cream of mushroom soup, chicken broth, salt, and pepper to the slow cooker.
4. Stir to combine all ingredients.
5. Cover and cook on low for 6-8 hours or until the rice is cooked through.

Nutritional Facts: (per serving, assuming 6 servings)

Calories: 300; Fat: 8g; Carbohydrates: 30g; Protein: 25g; Cholesterol: 60mg; Sodium: 700mg; Potassium: 550mg

10

Fish-Based Recipes

Tilapia and Rice Pilaf

PREP TIME:	COOKING TIME:	SERVINGS:
20 mins	4-6 hours	4-6

INGREDIENTS:

- 1 lb tilapia fillets, cubed
- 1 cup white rice, rinsed
- 2 cups mixed vegetables (peas, carrots, corn)
- 4 cups fish or chicken broth
- 1 tsp dried parsley
- Salt and pepper to taste

PORTION SIZES:

Small Dogs (under 20 pounds):

- Tilapia: 75 grams
- White rice: 40 grams
- Mixed vegetables (peas, carrots, corn): 60 grams
- Fish or chicken broth: 100 ml

Medium Dogs (20 - 50 pounds):

- Tilapia: 125 grams
- White rice: 65 grams
- Mixed vegetables (peas, carrots, corn): 100 grams
- Fish or chicken broth: 200 ml

Large Dogs (over 50 pounds):

- Tilapia: 200 grams
- White rice: 100 grams
- Mixed vegetables (peas, carrots, corn): 150 grams
- Fish or chicken broth: 300 ml

DIRECTIONS:

1. Place the cubed tilapia fillets, rinsed white rice, mixed vegetables, and fish or chicken broth in the slow cooker.
2. Add the dried parsley, salt, and pepper to the slow cooker.
3. Stir to combine all ingredients.
4. Cover and cook on low for 4-6 hours or until the tilapia is cooked through and the rice is tender.

Nutritional Facts: (per serving, assuming 6 servings)

Calories: 230; Fat: 2g; Carbohydrates: 30g; Protein: 25g; Cholesterol: 40mg; Sodium: 700mg; Potassium: 550mg

Haddock and Vegetable Casserole

PREP TIME:	COOKING TIME:	SERVINGS:
20 mins	4-6 hours	4-6

INGREDIENTS:

- 1 lb haddock fillets, cubed
- 2 cups sliced mushrooms
- 1 bell pepper, diced
- 1 can diced tomatoes, drained
- 4 cups fish or vegetable broth
- 1 tsp dried basil
- Salt and pepper to taste

PORTION SIZES:

Small Dogs (under 20 pounds):

- Haddock: 75 grams
- Sliced mushrooms: 40 grams
- Bell pepper: 20 grams
- Diced tomatoes: 20 grams
- Fish or vegetable broth: 100 ml

Medium Dogs (20 - 50 pounds):

- Haddock: 125 grams
- Sliced mushrooms: 65 grams
- Bell pepper: 30 grams
- Diced tomatoes: 30 grams
- Fish or vegetable broth: 200 ml

Large Dogs (over 50 pounds):

- Haddock: 200 grams
- Sliced mushrooms: 100 grams
- Bell pepper: 50 grams
- Diced tomatoes: 50 grams
- Fish or vegetable broth: 300 ml

DIRECTIONS:

1. Place the cubed haddock fillets, sliced mushrooms, diced bell pepper, diced tomatoes, and fish or vegetable broth in the slow cooker.
2. Add the dried basil, salt, and pepper to the slow cooker.
3. Stir to combine all ingredients.
4. Cover and cook on low for 4-6 hours or until the haddock is cooked through and the vegetables are tender.

Nutritional Facts: (per serving, assuming 6 servings)

Calories: 240; Fat: 2g; Carbohydrates: 20g; Protein: 25g; Cholesterol: 40mg; Sodium: 700mg; Potassium: 600mg

Trout and Lentil Soup

PREP TIME:	COOKING TIME:	SERVINGS:
20 mins	4-6 hours	4-6

INGREDIENTS:

- 1 lb trout fillets, skinless and boneless, cubed
- 1 cup dried green lentils, rinsed
- 2 carrots, peeled and sliced
- 4 cups fish or vegetable broth
- 1 tsp dried rosemary
- Salt and pepper to taste

PORTION SIZES:

Small Dogs (under 20 pounds):

- Trout: 75 grams
- Dried green lentils: 40 grams
- Carrots: 20 grams
- Fish or vegetable broth: 100 ml

Medium Dogs (20 -50 pounds):

- Trout: 125 grams
- Dried green lentils: 65 grams
- Carrots: 30 grams
- Fish or vegetable broth: 200 ml

Large Dogs (over 50 pounds):

- Trout: 200 grams
- Dried green lentils: 100 grams
- Carrots: 50 grams
- Fish or vegetable broth: 300 ml

DIRECTIONS:

1. Place the cubed trout fillets, rinsed green lentils, sliced carrots, and fish or vegetable broth In the slow cooker.
2. Add the dried rosemary, salt, and pepper to the slow cooker.
3. Stir to combine all ingredients.
4. Cover and cook on low for 4-6 hours or until the trout is cooked through and the lentils are tender.

Nutritional Facts: (per serving, assuming 6 servings)

Calories: 230; Fat: 3g; Carbohydrates: 25g; Protein: 20g; Cholesterol: 35mg; Sodium: 700mg; Potassium: 600mg

Mackerel and Vegetable Curry

PREP TIME:	COOKING TIME:	SERVINGS:
20 mins	4-6 hours	4-6

INGREDIENTS:

- 1 lb mackerel fillets, skinless and boneless, cubed
- 1 cup diced potatoes
- 1 cup diced carrots
- 1 bell pepper, diced
- 1 can of coconut milk
- 2 tbsp curry powder
- 4 cups fish or vegetable broth
- Salt and pepper to taste

PORTION SIZES:

Small Dogs (under 20 pounds):

- Mackerel: 75 grams
- Diced potatoes: 20 grams
- Diced carrots: 20 grams
- Bell pepper: 10 grams
- Coconut milk: 50 ml
- Curry powder: 1/2 tbsp
- Fish or vegetable broth: 100 ml

Medium Dogs (20 - 50 pounds):

- Mackerel: 125 grams
- Diced potatoes: 40 grams
- Diced carrots: 40 grams
- Bell pepper: 20 grams
- Coconut milk: 100 ml
- Curry powder: 1 tbsp
- Fish or vegetable broth: 200 ml

Large Dogs (over 50 pounds):

- Mackerel: 200 grams
- Diced potatoes: 65 grams
- Diced carrots: 65 grams
- Bell pepper: 30 grams
- Coconut milk: 150 ml
- Curry powder: 1 1/2 tbsp
- Fish or vegetable broth: 300 ml

DIRECTIONS:

1. Place the cubed mackerel fillets, diced potatoes, diced carrots, diced bell pepper, coconut milk, curry powder, and fish or vegetable broth in the slow cooker.
2. Stir to combine all ingredients.
3. Cover and cook on low for 4-6 hours or until the fish is cooked through and the vegetables are tender.
4. Serve over cooked rice or quinoa if desired.

Nutritional Facts: (per serving, assuming 6 servings)

Calories: 280; Fat: 15g; Carbohydrates: 15g; Protein: 25g; Cholesterol: 45mg; Sodium: 700mg; Potassium: 600mg

Haddock and Vegetable Chowder

PREP TIME:	COOKING TIME:	SERVINGS:
20 mins	4-6 hours	4-6

INGREDIENTS:

- 1 lb haddock fillets, skinless and boneless, cubed
- 2 potatoes, peeled and diced
- 1 cup sliced celery
- 1 cup corn kernels (fresh or frozen)
- 4 cups fish or vegetable broth
- 1 tsp dried thyme
- Salt and pepper to taste

PORTION SIZES:

Small Dogs (under 20 pounds):

- Haddock: 75 grams
- Potatoes: 20 grams
- Celery: 20 grams
- Corn kernels: 20 grams
- Fish or vegetable broth: 100 ml

Medium Dogs (20 -50 pounds):

- Haddock: 125 grams
- Potatoes: 40 grams
- Celery: 40 grams
- Corn kernels: 40 grams
- Fish or vegetable broth: 200 ml

Large Dogs (over 50 pounds):

- Haddock: 200 grams
- Potatoes: 65 grams
- Celery: 65 grams
- Corn kernels: 65 grams
- Fish or vegetable broth: 300 ml

DIRECTIONS:

1. Place the cubed haddock fillets, diced potatoes, sliced celery, and corn kernels in the slow cooker.
2. Add the fish or vegetable broth, dried thyme, salt, and pepper to the slow cooker.
3. Stir to combine all ingredients.
4. Cover and cook on low for 4-6 hours or until the haddock is cooked through and the vegetables are tender.

Nutritional Facts: (per serving, assuming 6 servings)

Calories: 220; Fat: 2g; Carbohydrates: 20g; Protein: 25g; Cholesterol: 40mg; Sodium: 700mg; Potassium: 600mg

Trout and Potato Casserole

PREP TIME:	**COOKING TIME:**	**SERVINGS:**
20 mins	4-6 hours	4-6

INGREDIENTS:

- 1 lb trout fillets, skinless and boneless, cubed
- 2 potatoes, peeled and diced
- 1 cup diced bell peppers (assorted colors)
- 1 cup sliced mushrooms
- 4 cups fish or vegetable broth
- 1 tsp dried basil
- Salt and pepper to taste

PORTION SIZES:

Small Dogs (under 20 pounds):

- Trout: 75 grams
- Potatoes: 20 grams
- Bell peppers: 20 grams
- Mushrooms: 20 grams
- Fish or vegetable broth: 100 ml

Medium Dogs (20 - 50 pounds):

- Trout: 125 grams
- Potatoes: 40 grams
- Bell peppers: 40 grams
- Mushrooms: 40 grams
- Fish or vegetable broth: 200 ml

Large Dogs (over 50 pounds):

- Trout: 200 grams
- Potatoes: 65 grams
- Bell peppers: 65 grams
- Mushrooms: 65 grams
- Fish or vegetable broth: 300 ml

DIRECTIONS:

1. Place the cubed trout fillets, diced potatoes, diced bell peppers, sliced mushrooms, and fish or vegetable broth in the slow cooker.
2. Add the dried basil, salt, and pepper to the slow cooker.
3. Stir to combine all ingredients.
4. Cover and cook on low for 4-6 hours or until the trout is cooked through and the potatoes are tender.

Nutritional Facts: (per serving, assuming 6 servings)

Calories: 230; Fat: 3g; Carbohydrates: 25g; Protein: 20g; Cholesterol: 35mg; Sodium: 700mg; Potassium: 600mg

Mackerel and Lentil Stew

PREP TIME:	COOKING TIME:	SERVINGS:
20 mins	4-6 hours	4-6

INGREDIENTS:

- 1 lb mackerel fillets, skinless and boneless, cubed
- 1 cup dried green lentils, rinsed
- 1 cup diced tomatoes
- 1 cup chopped spinach
- 4 cups fish or vegetable broth
- 1 tsp dried oregano
- Salt and pepper to taste

PORTION SIZES:

Small Dogs (under 20 pounds):

- Mackerel: 75 grams
- Dried green lentils: 40 grams
- Diced tomatoes: 40 grams
- Chopped spinach: 20 grams
- Fish or vegetable broth: 100 ml

Medium Dogs (20 - 50 pounds):

- Mackerel: 125 grams
- Dried green lentils: 65 grams
- Diced tomatoes: 65 grams
- Chopped spinach: 40 grams
- Fish or vegetable broth: 200 ml

Large Dogs (over 50 pounds):

- Mackerel: 200 grams
- Dried green lentils: 100 grams
- Diced tomatoes: 100 grams
- Chopped spinach: 50 grams
- Fish or vegetable broth: 300 ml

DIRECTIONS:

1. Place the cubed mackerel fillets, rinsed green lentils, diced tomatoes, chopped spinach, and fish or vegetable broth in the slow cooker.
2. Add the dried oregano, salt, and pepper to the slow cooker.
3. Stir to combine all ingredients.
4. Cover and cook on low for 4-6 hours or until the mackerel is cooked through and the lentils are tender.

Nutritional Facts: (per serving, assuming 6 servings)

Calories: 240; Fat: 4g; Carbohydrates: 25g; Protein: 25g; Cholesterol: 45mg; Sodium: 700mg; Potassium: 600mg

Cod and Vegetable Curry

PREP TIME:	COOKING TIME:	SERVINGS:
20 mins	4-6 hours	4-6

INGREDIENTS:

- 1 lb cod fillets, skinless and boneless, cubed
- 2 cups diced potatoes
- 1 cup diced carrots
- 1 cup diced bell peppers (assorted colors)
- 1 can of coconut milk
- 2 tbsp curry powder
- 4 cups fish or vegetable broth
- Salt and pepper to taste

PORTION SIZES:

Small Dogs (under 20 pounds):

- Cod: 75 grams
- Diced potatoes: 20 grams
- Diced carrots: 20 grams
- Diced bell peppers: 20 grams
- Coconut milk: 50 ml
- Curry powder: 1/2 tbsp
- Fish or vegetable broth: 100 ml

Medium Dogs (20 - 50 pounds):

- Cod: 125 grams
- Diced potatoes: 40 grams
- Diced carrots: 40 grams
- Diced bell peppers: 40 grams
- Coconut milk: 100 ml
- Curry powder: 1 tbsp
- Fish or vegetable broth: 200 ml

Large Dogs (over 50 pounds):

- Cod: 200 grams
- Diced potatoes: 65 grams
- Diced carrots: 65 grams
- Diced bell peppers: 65 grams
- Coconut milk: 150 ml
- Curry powder: 1.5 tbsp
- Fish or vegetable broth: 300 ml

DIRECTIONS:

1. Place the cubed cod fillets, diced potatoes, diced carrots, diced bell peppers, coconut milk, curry powder, and fish or vegetable broth in the slow cooker.
2. Stir to combine all ingredients.
3. Cover and cook on low for 4-6 hours or until the cod is cooked through and the vegetables are tender.
4. Serve over cooked rice or quinoa if desired.

Nutritional Facts: (per serving, assuming 6 servings)

Calories: 250; Fat: 10g; Carbohydrates: 20g; Protein: 20g; Cholesterol: 30mg; Sodium: 700mg; Potassium: 650mg

Sardine and Potato Stew

PREP TIME:	COOKING TIME:	SERVINGS:
20 mins	4-6 hours	4-6

INGREDIENTS:

- 2 cans sardines in olive oil, drained and flaked
- 2 potatoes, peeled and diced
- 2 carrots, peeled and sliced
- 4 cups fish or vegetable broth
- 1 tsp dried thyme
- Salt and pepper to taste

PORTION SIZES:

Small Dogs (under 20 pounds):

- Sardines: 50 grams
- Potatoes: 20 grams
- Carrots: 20 grams
- Fish or vegetable broth: 100 ml

Medium Dogs (20 - 50 pounds):

- Sardines: 75 grams
- Potatoes: 40 grams
- Carrots: 40 grams
- Fish or vegetable broth: 200 ml

Large Dogs (over 50 pounds):

- Sardines: 125 grams
- Potatoes: 65 grams
- Carrots: 65 grams
- Fish or vegetable broth: 300 ml

DIRECTIONS:

1. Place the flaked sardines, diced potatoes, sliced carrots, and fish or vegetable broth in the slow cooker.
2. Add the dried thyme, salt, and pepper to the slow cooker.
3. Stir to combine all ingredients.
4. Cover and cook on low for 4-6 hours or until the potatoes are tender.

Nutritional Facts: (per serving, assuming 6 servings)

Calories: 220; Fat: 8g; Carbohydrates: 20g; Protein: 15g; Cholesterol: 30mg; Sodium: 700mg; Potassium: 550mg

Cod and Vegetable Chowder

PREP TIME:	COOKING TIME:	SERVINGS:
20 mins	4-6 hours	4-6

INGREDIENTS:

- 1 lb cod fillets, skinless and boneless, cubed
- 2 potatoes, peeled and diced
- 2 carrots, peeled and sliced
- 4 cups fish or vegetable broth
- 1 cup corn kernels (fresh or frozen)
- Salt and pepper to taste

PORTION SIZES:

Small Dogs (under 20 pounds):

- Cod: 75 grams
- Potatoes: 20 grams
- Carrots: 20 grams
- Corn kernels: 20 grams
- Fish or vegetable broth: 100 ml

Medium Dogs (20 - 50 pounds):

- Cod: 125 grams
- Potatoes: 40 grams
- Carrots: 40 grams
- Corn kernels: 40 grams
- Fish or vegetable broth: 200 ml

Large Dogs (over 50 pounds):

- Cod: 200 grams
- Potatoes: 65 grams
- Carrots: 65 grams
- Corn kernels: 65 grams
- Fish or vegetable broth: 300 ml

DIRECTIONS:

1. Place the cubed cod fillets, diced potatoes, sliced carrots, and corn kernels in the slow cooker.
2. Add the fish or vegetable broth, salt, and pepper to the slow cooker.
3. Stir to combine all ingredients.
4. Cover and cook on low for 4-6 hours or until the cod is cooked through and the vegetables are tender.

Nutritional Facts: (per serving, assuming 6 servings)

Calories: 220; Fat: 1g; Carbohydrates: 30g; Protein: 25g; Cholesterol: 40mg; Sodium: 700mg; Potassium: 600mg

Chapter 4

SPECIAL DIETS AND DIETARY MODIFICATIONS

―――――――――

The comprehensive understanding of specialized diets and dietary modifications for slow cooker dog food involves an exploration of various factors, each tailored to meet the unique needs of individual dogs. These considerations span a range of health concerns, ranging from weight management and food allergies to specific medical conditions like renal disease, diabetes, and age-related issues.

One critical aspect of special diets revolves around weight management, where the focus lies on maintaining or achieving an optimal weight for the dog's health. In such cases, lean protein sources such as chicken breast or turkey serve as cornerstones, complemented by a generous inclusion of fiber-rich vegetables and fruits to promote satiety and digestive health. The careful balance of nutrients and portion control are key tenets in this approach, ensuring that calorie intake aligns with energy expenditure to support weight goals effectively.

Furthermore, addressing food allergies or sensitivities requires attention to ingredient selection, with a keen eye on avoiding known allergens such as wheat, dairy, and soy. Opting for alternative protein sources like beef, chicken, fish, lamb, or venison can circumvent potential triggers, while a deliberate avoidance of common allergenic ingredients mitigates the risk of adverse reactions. In cases of digestive issues, a gentle approach is warranted, focusing on easily digestible ingredients to alleviate discomfort. Cooked plain meats like chicken or turkey, supplemented by easily digestible carbohydrates such as rice or sweet potatoes, form the bedrock of this dietary modification, accompanied by bland vegetables like pumpkin or green beans to soothe sensitive stomachs.

Moreover, dogs grappling with renal or kidney disease necessitate a specialized diet characterized by low phosphorus and protein content to manage their condition effectively. Collaborating closely with a veterinarian is paramount in devising a tailored nutrition plan that incorporates low-phosphorus protein sources like egg whites or tofu, while strategically limiting high-phosphorus ingredients like organ meats or dairy products. The delicate balance between nutrient restriction and adequate nourishment is delicately orchestrated to support renal function and overall well-being.

Similarly, dogs diagnosed with diabetes necessitate a diet that regulates blood sugar levels and fosters weight management, emphasizing complex carbohydrates with a low glycemic index and lean protein sources to minimize glycemic fluctuations. Senior or geriatric dogs demand dietary adjustments that cater to their evolving needs as they age gracefully. This entails a focus on bolstering digestive health, supporting joint function, and nurturing cognitive vitality by incorporating key nutrients like omega-3 fatty acids, glucosamine, chondroitin, and antioxidants. Ingredients like fish or flaxseed oil provide essential omega-3 fatty acids to support cognitive function, while antioxidant-rich fruits and vegetables protect against age-related oxidative stress.

At the same time, increasing hydration levels is of greatest importance in improving overall health, particularly for dogs with a low water intake or those predisposed to urinary issues. Incorporating moisture-rich ingredients like broth, stock, or canned vegetables, coupled with ample water supplementation, fosters a state of hydration essential for optimal physiological function.

CATERING TO ALLERGIES AND FOOD SENSITIVITIES

Food allergies in dogs occur when their immune system mistakenly identifies certain proteins in their food as harmful invaders. When a dog with a predisposition to food allergies consumes a specific ingredient, their immune system reacts by producing antibodies, particularly immunoglobulin E (IgE) antibodies, to combat the perceived threat. Upon subsequent exposure to the allergen, these IgE antibodies trigger the release of histamine and other chemicals, leading to an inflammatory response. This response can manifest in various symptoms, such as itching, redness, swelling, gastrointestinal upset, ear infections, and skin issues.

While proteins like dairy and soy are common culprits for food allergies in dogs, any component of the diet has the potential to trigger an allergic reaction. It's important to recognize that food sensitivities may also occur, which may not involve the immune system but can lead to digestive discomfort and other mild symptoms due to difficulties in digesting or metabolizing certain ingredients. Identifying the specific allergen or sensitivity often requires a process of elimination through a specialized diet or consultation with a veterinarian.

Symptoms and Diagnosis

Food allergies and sensitivities in dogs often manifest in a variety of symptoms that can affect different parts of their body. Skin issues are a prominent sign, with dogs frequently exhibiting intense itching, leading to excessive scratching, licking, or chewing. This behavior can result in redness, irritation, hot spots, hair loss, and secondary skin infections. Gastrointestinal upset is another common symptom, presenting as diarrhea, vomiting, flatulence (gas), bloating, abdominal discomfort, and occasionally, the presence of blood or mucus in the stool. Some dogs may also experience a decreased appetite or weight loss due to digestive disturbances. Additionally, food allergies can contribute to recurring ear infections, characterized by redness, swelling, discharge, odor, and discomfort in the ears. These infections often stem from inflammation of the ear canal (otitis externa) secondary to the allergic response.

Diagnosing food allergies and sensitivities in dogs typically involves a comprehensive approach. An elimination diet trial is often employed, wherein the dog is fed a novel protein and carbohydrate source that they haven't been exposed to previously, while eliminating all other food sources, treats, and flavored medications. Observing any improvement in symptoms during the trial period and their recurrence upon reintroduction of the previous diet can strongly suggest a food allergy.

Designing Diets That Cater to Allergies and Food Sensitivities

Designing a diet tailored to cater to your dog's allergies and food sensitivities requires careful consideration and guidance from a veterinarian or veterinary nutritionist. Here are some steps to help you create a suitable diet plan:

1. **Identify Allergens:** Work with your veterinarian to pinpoint the specific ingredients causing your dog's allergic reactions. This may involve allergy testing, elimination diets, or observation of symptoms.
2. **Choose Hypoallergenic Ingredients:** Once allergens are identified, select hypoallergenic ingredients that are unlikely to trigger allergic reactions. These can include novel protein sources

such as venison, rabbit, duck, or fish, as well as novel carbohydrate sources like sweet potato, peas, or tapioca.

3. **Avoid Common Allergens:** Steer clear of ingredients commonly associated with food allergies in dogs, such as beef, chicken, dairy, eggs, soy, wheat, and corn.

4. **Select High-Quality Ingredients:** Opt for high-quality, easily digestible ingredients to support your dog's overall health and well-being. Look for dog food formulas that prioritize whole foods and limited ingredients and avoid artificial additives, preservatives, and fillers.

5. **Consider Commercial Hypoallergenic Diets:** There are commercially available hypoallergenic dog foods formulated specifically for dogs with food allergies or sensitivities. These diets typically feature novel protein and carbohydrate sources and may be supplemented with essential nutrients.

6. **Read Labels Carefully:** Always carefully read the labels of commercial dog foods to ensure they do not contain any ingredients your dog is allergic to. Be cautious of hidden allergens or cross-contamination during manufacturing.

7. **Monitor Symptoms:** Keep a close eye on your dog's symptoms and response to the new diet. If symptoms persist or worsen, consult with your veterinarian for further evaluation and adjustments to the diet plan.

8. **Consider Homemade or Raw Diets:** Some pet owners opt to prepare homemade or raw diets for their dogs with food allergies or sensitivities. If you choose this route, it's crucial to work with a veterinary nutritionist to ensure the diet is balanced, complete, and meets your dog's nutritional needs.

9. **Gradual Transition:** When transitioning to a new diet, do so gradually over several days to minimize digestive upset. Start by mixing a small amount of the new food with the old food and gradually increase the proportion of the new food while decreasing the old food.

Finally, veterinary examination, including physical assessment and possibly further tests to rule out other potential causes of allergy, is crucial. These may include blood tests, skin tests, or response to treatment with dietary changes or medication. Working closely with a veterinarian is essential to accurately diagnose and manage food allergies or sensitivities in dogs, as misdiagnosis or inadequate treatment can lead to ongoing discomfort and complications for your furry friend. Schedule regular check-ups with your veterinarian to monitor your dog's health, nutritional status, and any changes in symptoms. Adjustments to the diet may be necessary over time to address evolving needs or health concerns.

WEIGHT MANAGEMENT STRATEGIES

Effective weight management for dogs requires a detailed and comprehensive approach aimed at promoting healthy weight loss while ensuring overall well-being. Before initiating any weight loss program, it's essential to consult with a veterinarian who can assess your dog's current weight, body condition score (BCS), and overall health status. Based on this evaluation, realistic and achievable weight loss goals are established, typically aiming for a gradual reduction of 1-2% of body weight per week to ensure safe progress.

Diet plays a central role in weight management, with a focus on selecting high-quality, balanced commercial dog food formulated for weight loss or maintenance. These diets often have lower calorie content and higher fiber to promote satiety. Portion control is crucial, with precise measurement of food portions according to feeding guidelines provided by the manufacturer or veterinarian. Additionally, monitoring calorie intake carefully is essential to prevent overfeeding and ensure steady weight loss progress.

Regular exercise is another cornerstone of weight management, tailored to your dog's age, breed, size, and fitness level. Daily physical activity, such as brisk walks, jogging, or interactive play sessions, helps burn calories, maintain muscle mass, and support overall health.

Monitoring your dog's body condition score (BCS) regularly is important to track progress and adjust the weight management plan as needed. Visual and tactile assessments of your dog's waistline, ribs, and overall body shape are used to evaluate body composition, with the ideal being a defined waist and ribs that can be felt but not seen. In some cases, specialized weight loss diets or prescription diets may be recommended for dogs with significant obesity or obesity-related health issues, formulated to support weight loss while providing essential nutrients.

Behavioral factors that contribute to weight gain, such as begging or food stealing, should also be addressed through consistent feeding routines and the use of puzzle feeders or food-dispensing toys for mental stimulation. Regular follow-up appointments with the veterinarian are essential to monitor progress, adjust the weight management plan, and address any concerns or challenges encountered along the way.

RECIPES FOR DOGS WITH SPECIFIC HEALTH CONDITIONS

Dental Disease

Dental issues in dogs can range from gum disease to tooth decay. Meals prepared for this health condition have to be gentle on the teeth, soft, and easy to chew. Soft, moist foods that don't require much chewing can help relieve discomfort and prevent further dental problems. Recipes that feature tender meats, cooked vegetables, and soft textures can help ensure that dogs with dental sensitivity can still enjoy nutritious and delicious meals without worsening their condition.

1. **Chicken and Carrot Casserole:** This recipe features tender chicken and cooked carrots, which are gentle on the teeth and easy for dogs with dental problems to chew. The soft texture of the ingredients helps prevent discomfort while providing essential nutrients.

2. **Turkey and Butternut Squash**: Turkey is a lean protein source, and butternut squash can be cooked until soft, making it easier for dogs with dental issues to consume. This recipe offers a combination of protein and fiber-rich vegetables in a soft texture, ideal for dogs with dental sensitivity.

3. **Chicken and Tomato Soup:** Chicken soup provides a soft texture that's easy on the teeth, and the broth from the soup can help moisten dry kibble for easier chewing. Adding tomatoes to the soup provides essential vitamins and minerals while maintaining a soft consistency suitable for dogs with dental problems.

4. **Trout and Lentil Soup:** Trout is a soft fish, and when cooked in soup with lentils, it creates a nutritious and dental-friendly meal for dogs. This recipe offers a blend of protein and fiber in a soft texture, making it suitable for dogs with dental issues.

5. **Sardine and Potato Stew:** Sardines are a soft fish rich in omega-3 fatty acids, and potatoes can be cooked until tender, providing a gentle option for dogs with dental sensitivity. This stew offers a flavorful and nutritious meal with a soft texture that's easy for dogs with dental problems to enjoy.

The recipes listed have soft textures and easy-to-chew ingredients, making them ideal for dogs with dental issues. The presence of a variety of protein sources and vegetables in the meals provides essential nutrients needed for all-round nourishment.

Obesity

Obesity in dogs can lead to various health issues, including joint problems, diabetes, and heart disease. Therefore, it's essential to provide them with nutritious meals that support weight management. Recipes low in fat, moderate in carbohydrates, and high in lean protein and fiber are ideal for dogs dealing with obesity. These recipes should help them feel full while managing their weight.

1. **Chicken and Broccoli Casserole:** This recipe features lean chicken and fiber-rich broccoli, providing essential nutrients without excess calories. The low-fat content makes it suitable for dogs watching their weight.

2. **Turkey and Lentil Soup:** Turkey is a lean protein source, and lentils are high in fiber and low in fat, making this soup a satisfying and nutritious option for overweight dogs. The combination of protein and fiber helps keep dogs full without overloading them with calories.

3. **Chicken and Spinach Stew:** Lean chicken combined with nutrient-rich spinach offers a low-calorie yet filling meal option for dogs with obesity. The recipe provides essential nutrients while keeping fat content minimal.

4. **Trout and Lentil Soup:** Trout is a lean fish high in protein, and lentils provide fiber and essential nutrients without adding excessive calories. This soup is suitable for overweight dogs as it offers a balanced mix of protein and fiber with minimal fat content.

5. **Cod and Vegetable Curry:** Cod is a lean protein source, and vegetables in the curry provide fiber and essential nutrients while keeping the calorie count low. This recipe offers a flavorful and filling meal option for dogs managing their weight.

These slow cooker recipes prioritize lean protein sources, fiber-rich ingredients, and nutrient-dense vegetables to help dogs manage their weight effectively.

Ear Infection (Otitis Externa)

Ear infections are a common health issue in dogs, they can be painful and uncomfortable. Factors like bacteria, yeast, or allergies often cause it. Recipes rich in lean protein, omega-3 fatty acids, and immune-supportive nutrients can help reduce inflammation and promote ear health in dogs.

1. **Turkey and Butternut Squash:** Turkey is a lean protein source, and butternut squash is low in allergens and high in essential nutrients like vitamins A and C, which support immune function. This recipe avoids common allergens that contribute to ear infections while providing a nutritious meal option.

2. **Chicken and Tomato Soup:** Chicken soup provides a soft texture that's easy on the teeth, and the broth from the soup can help moisturize dry kibble for easier chewing. Tomatoes are rich in antioxidants and vitamins that support immune health, making this recipe beneficial for dogs prone to ear infections.

3. **Trout and Lentil Soup:** Trout is a lean fish high in protein and omega-3 fatty acids, which have anti-inflammatory properties that may help reduce inflammation associated with ear infections. Lentils provide fiber and essential nutrients without adding excessive calories, making this soup suitable for dogs with ear issues.

4. **Sardine and Potato Stew:** Sardines are rich in omega-3 fatty acids, which have anti-inflammatory properties that may help reduce inflammation in the ears. Potatoes provide carbohydrates for energy without aggravating allergies, making this stew a suitable option for dogs prone to ear infections.

5. **Haddock and Vegetable Chowder:** Haddock is a mild-flavored fish that's easy to digest, and vegetables in the chowder provide essential nutrients without common allergens that can contribute to ear issues. This recipe offers a comforting and nutritious meal option for dogs with sensitive ears.

Arthritis

Arthritis is a common condition in dogs, causing pain, stiffness, and reduced mobility. While medical treatment is essential, diet can play a significant role in managing arthritis symptoms and supporting joint health. Recipes rich in lean protein, omega-3 fatty acids, and anti-inflammatory ingredients can help alleviate pain and inflammation associated with arthritis.

1. **Chicken and Broccoli Casserole:** Chicken is a lean protein source that provides essential amino acids for muscle and joint health. Broccoli is rich in antioxidants and anti-inflammatory properties, making it beneficial for dogs with arthritis.

2. **Turkey and Lentil Soup:** Turkey is a lean protein source that provides essential nutrients for joint health. Lentils are high in fiber and contain anti-inflammatory properties, helping to reduce inflammation in arthritic joints.

3. **Trout and Lentil Soup:** Trout is rich in omega-3 fatty acids, which have anti-inflammatory properties that can help alleviate arthritis symptoms. Lentils provide fiber and essential nutrients without adding excessive calories, making this soup beneficial for dogs with arthritis.

4. **Sardine and Potato Stew:** Sardines are high in omega-3 fatty acids, which have been shown to reduce inflammation and improve joint health. Potatoes provide carbohydrates for energy without exacerbating arthritis symptoms, making this stew suitable for dogs with arthritis.

5. **Haddock and Vegetable Chowder:** Haddock is a mild-flavored fish that's easy to digest and rich in omega-3 fatty acids, which help reduce inflammation in arthritic joints. Vegetables in the chowder provide essential nutrients and antioxidants, supporting overall joint health.

Urinary Tract Infection

Urinary Tract Infections (UTIs) can be painful and uncomfortable for dogs, often caused by bacteria entering the urinary tract and leading to inflammation. Diet plays a crucial role in preventing and managing UTIs by promoting urinary tract health and reducing the risk of crystal formation. Recipes rich in lean protein, low in purines and oxalates, and containing ingredients with diuretic and anti-inflammatory properties can help support urinary tract health and reduce the likelihood of UTIs in dogs. By choosing recipes that consider their dietary needs, you can help prevent UTIs and support overall urinary tract health in your furry friend.

1. **Chicken and Carrot Casserole:** Chicken is a lean protein source that provides essential amino acids for overall health. Carrots are rich in antioxidants and contain natural diuretic properties that can help promote urinary tract health by increasing urine production and flushing out bacteria.

2. **Turkey and Butternut Squash:** Turkey is a lean protein source that's easy to digest and provides essential nutrients for overall health. Butternut squash is low in purines and oxalates, reducing the risk of crystal formation in the urinary tract and supporting urinary tract health.

3. **Chicken and Spinach Stew:** Chicken is a lean protein source that supports muscle and tissue health. Spinach is rich in vitamins and minerals, including potassium, which can help regulate urine pH and prevent the formation of urinary crystals that contribute to UTIs.

4. **Trout and Lentil Soup:** Trout is a high-quality protein source that's low in purines and oxalates, making it suitable for dogs prone to UTIs. Lentils are rich in fiber and contain beneficial nutrients that support urinary tract health, such as folate and magnesium.

5. **Sardine and Potato Stew:** Sardines are rich in omega-3 fatty acids, which have anti-inflammatory properties that can help reduce inflammation in the urinary tract and prevent UTIs. Potatoes provide carbohydrates for energy without contributing to urinary crystal formation, making this stew beneficial for dogs prone to UTIs.

Renal Disease

Renal (kidney) disease in dogs is a serious condition that requires careful dietary management to ensure the best possible quality of life. The kidneys play a critical role in filtering waste products from the blood, balancing electrolytes, and maintaining hydration. When the kidneys are compromised, it's essential to provide a diet that supports renal function and minimizes additional strain on these vital organs. For dogs with renal disease, suitable food should be low in phosphorus and protein, while being rich in high-quality, easily digestible proteins and beneficial fats. Additionally, sodium should be restricted to prevent hypertension and fluid retention, and the diet should include omega-3 fatty acids to help reduce inflammation and improve kidney health. Slow cooker recipes that are particularly suitable for dogs with renal disease include

1. **Turkey and Vegetable Stew:** Turkey is lower in phosphorus compared to other meats, making it easier on the kidneys. The inclusion of a variety of vegetables ensures the meal is rich in essential vitamins and minerals, without overloading the kidneys with excess protein. Additionally, the recipe can be prepared with low-sodium broth to further protect renal health.

2. **Chicken and Pumpkin Stew:** Chicken breast, being a low-fat protein source, helps in reducing the burden on the kidneys. Pumpkin adds fiber and moisture to the diet, which aids in digestion and can help maintain proper hydration levels. This recipe also allows for the addition of omega-3 fatty acids through fish oil supplements, which can reduce kidney inflammation and support overall kidney function.

3. **Beef and Sweet Potato Stew:** This is tailored for renal health by using lean cuts of beef, which are lower in phosphorus. Sweet potatoes provide a source of complex carbohydrates and fiber, essential for energy without overwhelming the kidneys with excess protein. This recipe can be enhanced by reducing the amount of beef and increasing the sweet potatoes and other vegetables to maintain a renal-friendly protein-to-carb ratio.

4. **Chicken and Carrot Casserole:** This recipe uses chicken as the primary protein source, known for being easy on the kidneys. Carrots are low in phosphorus and provide important antioxidants and vitamins. This recipe focuses on simplicity and ease of digestion, making it gentle on the kidneys while providing the necessary nutrients. Using low-sodium broth and incorporating omega-3 fatty acids can further enhance its suitability for dogs with renal issues.

5. **Turkey and Sweet Potato:** This recipe combines lean turkey meat with sweet potatoes, offering a balanced mix of protein and carbohydrates that are easier for dogs with kidney disease to process. The low phosphorus content of turkey, coupled with the high fiber and antioxidant properties of sweet potatoes, helps in managing renal function. This recipe is also conducive to the addition of renal-supportive supplements like omega-3 fatty acids.

Providing appropriate nutrition plays a vital role in managing various health conditions that dogs may face, including dental issues, obesity, ear infections, arthritis, urinary tract infections, and renal disease. Each of these conditions requires specific dietary considerations to support the dog's overall health, manage symptoms, and aid in recovery. By selecting recipes rich in lean proteins, essential nutrients, and ingredients with anti-inflammatory or immune-boosting properties, pet owners can contribute to their dog's well-being and quality of life. However, it's essential to remember that diet should complement veterinary care and medical treatment prescribed by professionals. Always consult with a veterinarian before making significant changes to a dog's diet, especially if they have a health condition requiring specialized nutrition. With proper attention to diet and veterinary guidance, pet owners can help their furry companions lead healthier and happier lives.

Chapter 5

MEAL PLANNING AND PORTION CONTROL

Meal planning and portion control are essential components of maintaining a healthy lifestyle, whether for ourselves or our furry companions. By carefully considering the nutritional needs and dietary requirements of individuals, we can create balanced meal plans that promote overall well-being. Portion control plays a pivotal role in ensuring that we consume the right amount of food to meet our energy needs without overindulging. In this chapter, we will explore the significance of meal planning and portion control, highlighting their benefits and providing practical insights into incorporating these practices into daily life. Whether you're looking to improve your eating habits or create balanced meal plans for your pets, understanding the principles of meal planning and portion control is key to achieving optimal health and vitality.

CREATING BALANCED MEAL PLANS

Designing a balanced meal plan for your dog is paramount for ensuring their overall health and well-being, much like it is for humans. When crafting a diet for your furry companion, it's crucial to consider a variety of factors to meet their nutritional requirements adequately.

First and foremost, protein stands as the cornerstone of a dog's diet. High-quality protein sources, such as lean meats like chicken, turkey, beef, and fish, should constitute a significant portion of their meals. These protein sources provide the necessary amino acids for muscle maintenance, immune function, and overall cellular health. It's essential to cook meat thoroughly to eliminate any potential bacterial contamination and ensure its safety for consumption by your pet. Additionally, eggs serve as an excellent protein source and can be included in your dog's diet, providing essential nutrients like vitamin A, riboflavin, and selenium.

Next, a variety of vegetables in your dog's meal plan is equally important. Vegetables offer essential vitamins, minerals, and fiber that contribute to overall health and digestion. Safe options include carrots, green beans, peas, sweet potatoes, and spinach. However, it's crucial to avoid feeding dogs onions, garlic, and mushrooms, as these can be toxic to them. Whether served raw or cooked, vegetables can be mixed with other components of the meal to create a balanced and nutritious diet for your pet. Carbohydrates provide dogs with a valuable source of energy. Opt for healthy carbohydrates like brown rice, quinoa, and oatmeal, which can be cooked and added to their meals. These grains not only provide energy but also offer additional nutrients and dietary fiber, which promotes digestive health. When incorporating carbohydrates into your dog's diet, ensure they are cooked thoroughly and served in appropriate portions to prevent any gastrointestinal issues.

Furthermore, fats play a crucial role in a dog's diet, supporting healthy skin and coat, as well as providing energy. Including healthy fats like those found in fish oil, flaxseed oil, or olive oil can enhance the nutritional value of your dog's meals. These fats can be added directly to their food or provided as a supplement, contributing to their overall well-being.

Calcium is essential for maintaining strong bones and teeth in dogs. Incorporating calcium-rich foods like yogurt, cheese, or cottage cheese into their diet can help meet their nutritional needs. Alternatively, you can use calcium supplements specifically formulated for dogs to ensure they receive an adequate amount of this vital mineral.

When it comes to feeding your dog a balanced diet, portion control is paramount. The appropriate portion size will vary depending on factors such as their size, age, and activity level. Consulting with your veterinarian to determine the ideal portion sizes for your dog ensures they receive the right amount of nutrients without overeating, which can lead to weight gain and associated health issues. Hydration is also crucial for your dog's health and well-being. Always ensure they have access to fresh, clean water at all times to prevent dehydration and promote proper digestion.

DETERMINING PORTION SIZES

Determining portion sizes for your dog when preparing wholesome homemade meals is a critical aspect of their overall health and well-being. Unlike commercial dog foods, which often provide feeding guidelines based on the dog's weight, homemade meals require a more personalized approach. There are several factors to consider when determining the appropriate portion sizes for your furry friend, including their size, age, activity level, metabolism, specific dietary requirements, and any underlying health conditions they may have. Consulting with your veterinarian is the first step in this process, as they can offer tailored recommendations based on your dog's individual needs and circumstances.

One of the primary considerations in determining portion sizes for homemade meals is your dog's size. Larger dogs typically require larger portion sizes to meet their energy needs, while smaller dogs may need smaller portions. However, it's essential to consider factors beyond just size, such as breed, body composition, and metabolism. For example, a small but highly active breed may require more calories than a larger, more sedentary dog. Additionally, puppies and senior dogs have different nutritional requirements than adult dogs, so their portion sizes will need to be adjusted accordingly.

Age is another crucial factor to consider when determining portion sizes for homemade meals. Puppies have higher energy requirements than adult dogs due to their rapid growth and development. As a result, they may need more frequent meals and larger portion sizes to support their growth. Conversely, senior dogs may have lower energy needs and may require smaller portion sizes to prevent weight gain and obesity. It's essential to adjust portion sizes as your dog ages to ensure they're receiving the appropriate amount of nutrients for their life stage.

Activity level plays a significant role in determining portion sizes for dogs. Active dogs who engage in regular exercise, such as agility training, hiking, or playing fetch, burn more calories and may require larger portion sizes to fuel their activity. On the other hand, less active dogs, such as couch potatoes or senior pets, may need smaller portion sizes to prevent weight gain and maintain a healthy body condition. It's crucial to assess your dog's activity level accurately and adjust portion sizes accordingly to meet their energy needs.

Metabolism varies from dog to dog and can impact how efficiently they digest and utilize nutrients from their food. Some dogs have faster metabolisms and may require more calories to maintain their weight, while others have slower metabolisms and may be more prone to weight gain. Factors such as breed, age, and overall health can influence metabolism. Dogs with medical conditions such as thyroid issues or diabetes may have unique dietary requirements, and their portion sizes may need to be carefully monitored and adjusted under the guidance of a veterinarian. Specific dietary requirements or preferences should also be taken into account when determining portion sizes for homemade meals. For example, some dogs may have food allergies or sensitivities that require them to avoid certain ingredients, while others may have dietary restrictions due to medical conditions such as kidney disease or pancreatitis. Additionally, some dogs may prefer certain types of food over others, and their portion sizes may need to be adjusted accordingly to ensure they receive a balanced diet that meets their nutritional needs.

Monitoring your dog's weight and body condition is essential for ensuring they're receiving the appropriate portion sizes for their needs. Ideally, you should be able to feel your dog's ribs without them being too prominent or hidden beneath a layer of fat. If your dog is gaining or losing weight unintentionally, it may be a sign that their portion sizes need to be adjusted. Regular weigh-ins and body condition assessments can help you track your dog's progress and make any necessary changes to their diet.

In addition to considering portion sizes, it's essential to ensure that homemade meals provide a balanced and nutritionally complete diet for your dog. This includes incorporating a variety of high-quality protein sources, healthy carbohydrates, essential fats, vitamins, and minerals into their meals. Protein is particularly important for dogs, as it provides the building blocks for muscle maintenance, immune function, and overall cellular health. Good sources of protein include lean meats such as chicken, turkey, beef, and fish, as well as eggs and dairy products. Carbohydrates provide dogs with a valuable source of energy and should include healthy options like brown rice, quinoa, and sweet potatoes. Fats are necessary for healthy skin and coat, as well as providing energy, and should include sources like fish oil, flaxseed oil, or olive oil.

ESTABLISHING FEEDING SCHEDULE

Establishing a feeding schedule for your dog is essential for maintaining their health, promoting proper digestion, and managing their weight. A consistent feeding routine provides structure and helps prevent overeating or underfeeding. Here's a comprehensive guide to help you establish a feeding schedule tailored to your dog's needs

1. **Consult Your Vet:** Before establishing a feeding schedule, consult with your veterinarian to determine the appropriate number of meals and portion sizes for your dog based on their age, size, breed, activity level, and any specific dietary requirements or health conditions they may have.
2. **Select the Number of Meals:** Dogs typically thrive on either two meals per day or three smaller meals, depending on their age, size, and lifestyle. Puppies, senior dogs, and dogs with certain health conditions may benefit from three meals spaced throughout the day to maintain stable blood sugar levels and provide sustained energy. Adult dogs usually do well with two meals, one in the morning and one in the evening.

3. **Establish a Routine:** Choose specific times for feeding your dog and stick to them consistently. Dogs thrive on routine, so feeding them at the same times each day helps regulate their metabolism and digestion. Avoid free-feeding, where food is left out all day for your dog to eat whenever they please, as this can lead to overeating and weight gain.

4. **Morning Meal:** If you're feeding your dog twice a day, the morning meal is typically served shortly after you wake up. This meal provides the energy your dog needs to start their day and fuel any morning activities or exercise. Aim to feed your dog at least 30 minutes to an hour before any vigorous activity to prevent stomach upset.

5. **Evening Meal:** The evening meal should be served several hours before bedtime to allow your dog time to digest their food properly before settling down for the night. Feeding your dog too close to bedtime can increase the risk of digestive issues like indigestion or acid reflux. Aim to feed your dog their evening meal at least 2-3 hours before bedtime.

6. **Spacing Meals:** If you're feeding your dog three meals a day, aim to space them out evenly throughout the day. For example, you could feed your dog breakfast in the morning, lunch in the early afternoon, and dinner in the early evening. This schedule helps prevent hunger between meals and provides a steady source of energy throughout the day.

7. **Monitor Meal Times:** Pay attention to your dog's behavior and appetite to determine if the chosen meal times are suitable for them. Some dogs may prefer to eat earlier or later than others, so be flexible and adjust the schedule as needed to accommodate their preferences.

8. **Consider Treats and Snacks:** If you offer treats or snacks to your dog throughout the day, factor these into their overall daily caloric intake. Treats should make up no more than 10% of your dog's daily calories to prevent overfeeding. Consider using treats as rewards for training or as a way to provide mental stimulation for your dog.

9. **Hydration:** Always ensure your dog has access to fresh, clean water at all times, especially during meal times. Proper hydration is essential for digestion and overall health.

10. **Special Considerations:** Some dogs may have special dietary needs or health conditions that require a modified feeding schedule. For example, diabetic dogs may need to eat smaller, more frequent meals to help regulate their blood sugar levels. Always follow your veterinarian's recommendations when establishing a feeding schedule for a dog with specific health concerns.

Chapter 6

INCORPORATING SUPPLEMENTS

UNDERSTANDING NUTRITIONAL SUPPLEMENTS

Nutritional supplements have become popular in human health and wellness, promising an array of benefits ranging from improved immunity and energy levels to enhanced cognitive function and overall vitality. This trend has extended to pet care, with an abundance of supplements now available specifically tailored to meet the unique nutritional needs of canine friends. However, among numerous options lining store shelves and online marketplaces, pet owners are often left with questions and uncertainties regarding the efficacy, safety, and necessity of these supplements for their furry companions. Understanding nutritional supplements involves demystifying common misconceptions, and empowering pet owners to make informed decisions about supplementing their dogs' diets.

What role do nutritional supplements play in supporting canine health and well-being? While the primary function of a dog's diet is to provide essential nutrients necessary for the growth, development, and maintenance of bodily functions, nutritional supplements are designed to complement this diet by supplying additional vitamins, minerals, antioxidants, and other bioactive compounds that may be lacking or insufficient in the dog's regular food. These supplements are often marketed as a means of addressing specific health concerns or optimizing overall health, offering a convenient and targeted approach to filling nutritional gaps and promoting optimal wellness in dogs of all ages and breeds.

One of the key considerations in understanding nutritional supplements is recognizing the diverse array of products available and their respective benefits and potential drawbacks. From multivitamins and mineral complexes to specialized formulations targeting joint health, skin and coat condition, digestive health, and cognitive function, the supplement market for dogs is vast and varied. Each product is formulated with specific ingredients chosen for their purported benefits, whether it be glucosamine and chondroitin for joint support, omega-3 fatty acids for skin and coat health, or probiotics for digestive balance. However, it is essential to approach these supplements with a critical eye, recognizing that not all products are created equal, and not all claims may be supported by scientific evidence.

Indeed, one of the challenges in navigating the world of nutritional supplements is discerning fact from fiction and understanding the limitations of available research. While some supplements have been extensively studied and demonstrated clear benefits in clinical trials, others may lack robust scientific evidence to support their efficacy or safety. In many cases, the efficacy of a supplement may depend on factors such as the quality and bioavailability of its ingredients, the dosage and frequency of administration, and the individual dog's unique health status and nutritional needs. As such, pet owners are encouraged to consult with their veterinarian before introducing any new supplement into their dog's diet, ensuring that it aligns with their dog's specific health goals and does not pose any risk of adverse effects or interactions with existing medications or conditions.

Another important aspect of understanding nutritional supplements is recognizing that they are not a substitute for a balanced and nutritious diet. While supplements can play a valuable role in addressing specific health concerns or supporting overall wellness, they should ideally complement a high-quality commercial dog food or homemade diet that provides essential nutrients in appropriate proportions. Moreover, reliance on supplements to compensate for deficiencies in the primary diet may mask underlying issues with diet quality or nutrient bioavailability, potentially exacerbating health problems in the long run. Therefore, pet owners are encouraged to prioritize the quality and nutritional adequacy of their dog's regular diet before considering supplementation as a secondary measure.

RECOMMENDED SUPPLEMENTS FOR CANINE HEALTH

Several supplements can support canine health, providing additional nutrients to promote overall well-being. Here are some recommended supplements for canine health:

1. **Omega-3 Fatty Acids:** Promotes skin and coat health, reduces inflammation, supports joint health, and may enhance cognitive function. Look for supplements containing EPA and DHA.

2. **Glucosamine and Chondroitin:** Supports joint health and mobility by maintaining cartilage integrity and elasticity, particularly beneficial for senior dogs or those with arthritis.

3. **Probiotics:** Supports digestive health and strengthen the immune system by maintaining a healthy balance of gut flora, reducing the risk of gastrointestinal issues, especially helpful for dogs with sensitive stomachs or on antibiotics.

4. **Antioxidants:** Neutralizes harmful free radicals, protects cells from oxidative damage, and reduces the risk of chronic diseases. Includes vitamins C and E, selenium, and beta-carotene.

5. **Multivitamins:** Fills nutritional gaps in the diet, particularly beneficial for dogs with specific dietary restrictions or health conditions and supports overall health.

6. **Digestive Enzymes:** Aids digestion and nutrient absorption, especially helpful for dogs with pancreatic insufficiency or digestive disorders.

7. **Coenzyme Q10 (CoQ10):** Supports heart health and cellular energy production, beneficial for senior dogs or those with heart conditions.

8. **Joint Support Formulas:** Contains glucosamine, chondroitin, MSM, hyaluronic acid, and turmeric to support joint health, and mobility, and reduce inflammation.

9. **Calcium:** Essential for bone health and muscle function, particularly important for growing puppies, pregnant or lactating dogs, and senior dogs with bone density issues.

10. **Vitamin D:** Facilitates calcium absorption, crucial for bone health and immune function.

11. **Vitamin E:** Acts as an antioxidant, supports immune function, and promotes healthy skin and coat.

12. **B-vitamins:** Including B1 (thiamine), B2 (riboflavin), B3 (niacin), B6 (pyridoxine), and B12 (cobalamin), essential for energy metabolism, nerve function, and overall health.

13. **Iron:** Supports red blood cell production and oxygen transport, essential for preventing anemia.

14. **Zinc:** Supports immune function, skin health, wound healing, and overall growth and development.

15. **Magnesium:** Supports bone health, muscle function, and nerve transmission.

16. **Selenium:** Acts as an antioxidant, supports thyroid function, and plays a role in immune response.

17. **L-carnitine:** Supports energy metabolism and cardiovascular health.

18. **Fiber:** Supports digestive health and regulates bowel movements, beneficial for dogs with gastrointestinal issues such as constipation or diarrhea.

19. **Methylsulfonylmethane (MSM):** Provides sulfur, which supports joint health, reduces inflammation, and promotes tissue repair.

20. **Hyaluronic Acid:** Supports joint health and mobility by lubricating joints and promoting cartilage health.

GUIDELINES FOR SAFE AND EFFECTIVE SUPPLEMENT USE

When incorporating supplements into your dog's routine, it's essential to prioritize safety and effectiveness. Here are some guidelines to ensure safe and effective supplement use for your furry companion:

1. **Consult with Your Veterinarian:** Before adding any supplements to your dog's diet, consult with your veterinarian. They can provide personalized recommendations based on your dog's specific needs, health status, and any existing medical conditions. Your vet can also advise on the appropriate type, dosage, and duration of supplementation for your dog.

2. **Choose High-Quality Supplements:** Select supplements from reputable brands that adhere to stringent quality control standards. Look for supplements that have undergone third-party testing for purity, potency, and safety. Avoid supplements with unnecessary fillers, additives, or artificial ingredients.

3. **Read and Follow Dosage Instructions:** Follow the manufacturer's dosage instructions carefully to ensure your dog receives the correct amount of supplement. Avoid exceeding the recommended dosage, as this can lead to adverse effects or toxicity. If in doubt, consult your veterinarian for guidance on dosing.

4. **Monitor for Adverse Effects:** Keep an eye out for any adverse effects or changes in your dog's behavior, appetite, or health after starting a new supplement. Common adverse effects may include gastrointestinal upset, allergic reactions, or changes in urine or stool. If you notice any concerning symptoms, discontinue the supplement and consult your veterinarian.

5. **Give with Food:** Some supplements are best given with food to enhance absorption and minimize gastrointestinal upset. Follow the manufacturer's instructions regarding whether to

administer the supplement with or without food. If your dog experiences stomach upset, try giving the supplement with a meal or adjusting the dosage.

6. **Be Patient and Consistent:** It may take time to see noticeable results from supplements, especially for long-term health benefits like joint support or skin and coat improvement. Be patient and consistent with supplement use, following the recommended dosage and administration schedule as directed.

7. **Rotate Supplements Carefully:** Avoid overloading your dog with multiple supplements at once, as this can increase the risk of nutrient imbalances or toxicity. If your dog requires multiple supplements, rotate them carefully to ensure they receive a balanced and varied diet. Consult with your veterinarian to develop a supplementation plan tailored to your dog's needs.

8. **Consider Individual Needs:** Every dog is unique, and their nutritional requirements may vary based on factors like age, breed, size, activity level, and health status. Consider your dog's individual needs and health goals when selecting supplements. Your veterinarian can provide personalized recommendations to address specific concerns or deficiencies.

9. **Regularly Reassess:** Periodically reassess your dog's supplement regimen to ensure it remains appropriate and effective. As your dog's health and nutritional needs change over time, adjustments to supplementation may be necessary. Consult with your veterinarian for guidance on modifying or discontinuing supplements as needed.

10. **Integrate Supplements into a Balanced Diet:** Supplements should complement, not replace, a balanced and nutritionally complete diet for your dog. Focus on providing a high-quality, balanced diet tailored to your dog's specific needs, and use supplements as needed to fill any nutritional gaps or support specific health goals.

By following these guidelines, you can ensure safe and effective supplement use for your dog, supporting their overall health and well-being.

Chapter 7

TRANSITIONING TO HOMEMADE MEALS

Transitioning to homemade meals for your dog can be a rewarding journey that offers numerous benefits, including greater control over ingredients, customization of nutrients to meet individual needs, and potentially improved health and well-being. Whether motivated by concerns over commercial pet food quality, specific dietary requirements, or simply a desire to provide a more natural and wholesome diet, the transition process requires careful planning, patience, and a gradual approach. By understanding the key considerations, such as nutritional balance, portion control, and monitoring progress, dog owners can successfully navigate the transition to homemade meals and provide their furry companions with a diet that supports their overall health and vitality.

GRADUAL TRANSITIONING PROCESS

Transitioning your dog to a homemade meal necessitates a thoughtful and gradual approach to ensure a smooth transition and minimize digestive issues. The process involves several crucial steps aimed at providing your furry companion with a balanced and nutritionally complete diet while also considering their individual needs, preferences, and health status.

Consulting with your veterinarian is the first and most crucial step in this process, as they can offer personalized recommendations based on your dog's specific nutritional requirements, age, breed, size, and any existing health conditions. Veterinary guidance ensures that your homemade meal plan meets your dog's needs and supports their overall health and well-being.

Once you have the green light from your veterinarian, the next step is to research and plan your dog's homemade meals meticulously. Look for recipes and ingredients that provide a balanced combination of high-quality protein sources, healthy carbohydrates, fats, vitamins, and minerals. Aim to include a variety of ingredients to ensure your dog receives a wide range of nutrients. Consider factors such as your dog's taste preferences, food sensitivities or allergies, and any dietary restrictions when selecting recipes and ingredients. It's essential to strike a balance between nutritional adequacy and palatability to ensure your dog enjoys their meals while still meeting their dietary needs.

When initiating the transition to homemade meals, it's crucial to start slowly and gradually introduce the new food into your dog's diet while still feeding their regular food. Begin by mixing small amounts of homemade food with their regular food to allow your dog's digestive system time to adjust. Monitor your dog closely for any signs of digestive upset, such as vomiting, diarrhea, or changes in appetite or stool quality. If you notice any adverse reactions, slow down the transition process or consult with your veterinarian for guidance on how to proceed. As your dog becomes accustomed to homemade food, gradually increase the proportion of homemade food in their meals while decreasing the amount of their regular food. This gradual transition allows your dog's digestive system to gradually adapt to the new diet. Monitor your dog's response closely and adjust the transition pace as needed based on their tolerance and digestive health. It's essential to proceed at a pace that is comfortable for your dog and minimizes the risk of digestive upset.

Throughout the transition process, maintain consistency in your dog's feeding routine and meal composition. Consistency is key to preventing digestive upset and ensuring that your dog receives a balanced and nutritionally complete diet. Establish a regular feeding schedule and stick to it, providing meals at the same times each day. Consistency also helps your dog adjust to their new diet more smoothly and reduces the likelihood of food aversions or behavioral issues.

As your dog fully transitions to homemade meals, continue to monitor their overall health, weight, and nutritional status. Consider joining online forums or communities dedicated to homemade dog food to share experiences, ask questions, and learn from others. By staying informed and connected, you can ensure that your dog receives the best possible care and nutrition.

OVERCOMING COMMON CHALLENGES

Transitioning your dog to a homemade meal can be a rewarding but challenging process. It is a process that requires patience, careful planning, and flexibility. While the goal is to provide your furry companion with a nutritious and balanced diet, several common challenges may arise during the transition process.

Digestive Upset

One of the most common challenges during the transition to a homemade meal is digestive upset, such as vomiting, diarrhea, or gastrointestinal discomfort. To minimize digestive issues, start the transition slowly by gradually introducing small amounts of homemade food into your dog's diet while still feeding their regular food. Monitor your dog closely for any signs of digestive upset and adjust the transition pace as needed. If digestive issues persist, consult with your veterinarian for guidance on how to address them effectively.

Food Aversion

Some dogs may be resistant to trying new foods, especially if they are accustomed to a particular diet or have strong preferences. To overcome food aversion, gradually introduce new ingredients and flavors into your dog's meals, mixing them with familiar foods to make the transition more appealing. Be patient and persistent, offering small tastes of the new food and gradually increasing the amount over time. Positive reinforcement, such as praise or treats, can also encourage your dog to try new foods and make the transition smoother.

Nutritional Imbalances

Ensuring that your homemade meals provide all the essential nutrients your dog needs can be challenging. To overcome nutritional imbalances, research recipes, and ingredients carefully to ensure they meet your dog's nutritional requirements. Consider consulting with a veterinary nutritionist or using reputable resources to formulate balanced meal plans tailored to your dog's specific needs. Regularly monitor your dog's overall health and well-being and consult with your veterinarian if you have any concerns about nutritional adequacy or deficiencies.

Palatability Issues

Some homemade recipes may not be as palatable to your dog as commercial dog food, leading to reluctance or refusal to eat. To address palatability issues, experiment with different ingredients, flavors, and textures to find what your dog enjoys. Adding natural flavor enhancers, such as low-sodium broth or bone broth, can make homemade meals more appealing to picky eaters. Avoiding sudden changes in diet and maintaining a consistent feeding routine can also help encourage your dog to eat their homemade meals.

Time and Preparation

Preparing homemade meals for your dog can be time-consuming and require careful planning, especially if you're cooking from scratch or using fresh ingredients. To overcome time and preparation challenges, consider batch cooking and freezing portions of homemade meals for future use. Invest in time-saving tools and kitchen appliances, such as slow cookers or food processors, to streamline the cooking process. Alternatively, explore pre-made or freeze-dried commercial options that offer the convenience of homemade meals without the hassle of preparation.

Cost Considerations

Homemade meals for your dog may be more expensive than commercial dog food, depending on the ingredients and recipes you choose. To manage cost considerations, plan your dog's meals budget carefully and explore cost-effective options for sourcing ingredients. Consider buying in bulk, using seasonal produce, or incorporating budget-friendly protein sources, such as eggs or legumes, into your dog's meals. Additionally, prioritize quality over quantity when it comes to ingredients, focusing on nutrient-dense foods that offer the most nutritional value for your money.

Consult with a Veterinarian

If you encounter challenges during the transition process or have concerns about your dog's health or nutrition, don't hesitate to consult with your veterinarian for guidance and support. Your vet can offer personalized recommendations, troubleshoot any issues you may encounter, and provide reassurance and encouragement as you navigate the transition to a homemade diet. With their expertise and guidance, you can overcome challenges and ensure that your dog receives the best possible care and nutrition.

MONITORING PROGRESS AND ADJUSTING AS NEEDED

Monitoring your dog's progress and adjusting as needed during the transition to a homemade meal is a vital part of ensuring their health and well-being. Observing your dog's eating behavior, appetite, and digestive health provides invaluable insights into how well they are adapting to the new diet. Positive signs, such as a healthy appetite and eagerness to consume homemade food, indicate a smooth transition process. Conversely, any signs of digestive upset, such as vomiting, diarrhea, gastrointestinal discomfort, or reluctance to eat may signal the need for adjustments in the transition plan.

Regularly assessing your dog's overall health is equally important. Pay attention to changes in energy levels, coat condition, and weight to gauge the effectiveness of the new diet. Improved vitality, a shinier coat, brighter eyes, and increased mobility are positive indicators that your dog is thriving on their homemade meals. Conversely, if you notice lethargy, dull coat, weight loss, or changes in behavior, it may be necessary to reassess the diet and make adjustments to address any deficiencies or imbalances.

Adjusting portion sizes is one way to tailor your dog's homemade meals to their individual needs. Factors such as age, size, activity level, and weight management goals should be taken into consideration when determining the appropriate portion sizes for your dog. Monitor your dog's body condition score and weight regularly to ensure they are maintaining a healthy weight. If your dog is gaining or losing weight unintentionally, adjusting their portion sizes accordingly can help achieve and maintain an ideal body condition.

Modifying the composition of your dog's homemade meals can also contribute to their overall health and well-being. Experiment with different ingredients, flavors, and textures to find what works best for your dog. Consider rotating protein sources, incorporating a variety of fruits and vegetables, and adding supplements as needed to ensure your dog receives a balanced and nutritionally complete diet. For example, if your dog has specific dietary restrictions or preferences, such as food sensitivities or allergies, you may need to tailor their meals accordingly.

Chapter 8
STORAGE AND SERVING SUGGESTIONS

STORAGE OF HOMEMADE DOG FOOD

P roper storage of homemade dog food is required to maintain its freshness, nutritional integrity, and safety for your dog. When preparing homemade meals for your dog, it is essential to follow specific guidelines to ensure that the food remains safe and nutritious for consumption.

One of the primary considerations is refrigeration. After preparing or serving homemade dog food, it should be promptly refrigerated to slow down bacterial growth and preserve its freshness. Utilizing airtight containers or resealable bags can help maintain the food's quality and prevent contamination. Refrigerated homemade dog food should be stored at a consistent temperature of 40°F (4°C) or below, as this inhibits the growth of harmful bacteria that could lead to foodborne illness. It's advisable to use a refrigerator thermometer to monitor the temperature regularly and ensure it remains within the safe range. Additionally, homemade dog food should be stored away from the refrigerator door, as temperature fluctuations in this area can compromise its quality and safety.

Another crucial aspect of storing homemade dog food is proper labeling with best-before dates. Labeling containers with the date of preparation and best-before date allows pet owners to track the freshness of the food and ensure timely consumption. Homemade dog food typically has a shorter shelf life compared to commercial pet food, so it's essential to use it within a few days to a week, depending on the ingredients used and storage conditions. Consuming homemade dog food past its use-by date can increase the risk of spoilage and foodborne illness, so it's crucial to adhere to these guidelines to maintain your pet's health and safety.

Freezing is another option for storing homemade dog food, especially if prepared in large batches or to extend its shelf life. Before freezing, divide the homemade food into individual servings or portions and place them in airtight freezer-safe containers or freezer bags. Proper packaging helps prevent freezer burn and maintain the food's quality during storage. Labeling frozen homemade dog food with the date of preparation allows pet owners to keep track of its freshness and ensures timely consumption. When stored properly, frozen homemade dog food can be kept for several months, depending on the ingredients used and storage conditions. Thawing frozen homemade dog food safely is essential to preserve its quality and prevent bacterial growth. It's recommended to thaw frozen dog food overnight in the refrigerator or cold water for quicker thawing. Avoid thawing homemade dog food at room temperature or using the microwave, as these methods can promote bacterial growth and compromise food safety.

In addition to proper storage techniques, maintaining good hygiene practices when handling and serving homemade dog food is essential to prevent cross-contamination and foodborne illness. Washing hands thoroughly with soap and water before and after handling dog food helps reduce the risk of spreading harmful bacteria. Regularly cleaning food preparation surfaces and utensils with hot, soapy water minimizes the risk of contamination. It's also crucial to avoid using the same utensils or containers for raw and cooked ingredients to prevent cross-contamination. By practicing good hygiene habits, pet owners can ensure the safety and quality of homemade dog food for their furry companions.

Inspecting homemade dog food for signs of spoilage before serving is another critical step in maintaining its safety and quality. Pet owners should routinely check for any unusual odors, mold growth, or changes in texture or appearance, as these may indicate spoilage. If any abnormalities are detected, homemade dog food should be discarded immediately to prevent the risk of foodborne illness. Regularly inspecting homemade dog food for signs of spoilage helps ensure that pets are consuming safe and nutritious meals that support their health and well-being.

SERVING SIZES AND RECOMMENDATIONS

Determining appropriate serving sizes and providing recommendations for homemade dog food is crucial for ensuring that your furry companion receives the right balance of nutrients and maintains a healthy weight. Serving sizes should be tailored to your dog's individual needs, taking into account factors such as age, size, breed, activity level, and any specific dietary requirements or health conditions. The guidelines provided help you determine serving sizes and make recommendations for homemade dog food.

1. **Calculate Caloric Needs:** Start by calculating your dog's daily caloric needs based on factors such as their weight, age, and activity level. You can use online calculators or consult with your veterinarian to determine the appropriate caloric intake for your dog. Knowing your dog's caloric needs provides a baseline for determining serving sizes and adjusting portion sizes as needed.

2. **Consider Nutritional Requirements:** Homemade dog food should be nutritionally balanced to meet your dog's dietary requirements. Ensure that homemade meals contain a balanced combination of high-quality protein sources, healthy carbohydrates, fats, vitamins, and minerals. Consult with a veterinary nutritionist or use reputable resources to formulate balanced meal plans tailored to your dog's specific needs. Pay attention to recommended daily allowances for key nutrients, such as protein, fat, fiber, vitamins, and minerals, and adjust serving sizes accordingly to meet these requirements.

3. **Monitor Weight and Body Condition:** Regularly monitor your dog's weight and body condition to assess whether serving sizes are appropriate and adjust accordingly. Use body condition scoring systems, such as the 1-9 scale, to evaluate your dog's body composition and ensure they maintain a healthy weight. If your dog is gaining or losing weight unintentionally, adjust serving sizes to help them achieve and maintain an ideal body condition.

4. **Assess Activity Level:** Take your dog's activity level into account when determining serving sizes. Dogs with higher activity levels or those engaged in strenuous activities, such as agility training or working dogs, may require more calories to support their energy needs. Conversely, dogs with lower activity levels or those who are less active may require fewer calories to prevent weight gain.

5. **Adjust Portions Gradually:** When making changes to serving sizes, do so gradually to allow your dog's digestive system time to adjust. Monitor your dog's response closely and make adjustments as needed based on their appetite, energy levels, and overall well-being. Avoid sudden changes in portion sizes, as this can lead to digestive upset or weight changes.

6. **Feed Multiple Meals:** Consider dividing your dog's daily food allowance into multiple smaller meals throughout the day to help regulate their appetite, prevent overeating, and maintain stable energy levels. Feeding smaller, more frequent meals can also help prevent digestive issues and promote better digestion and nutrient absorption.

Large Breed Dogs (Over 50 lbs)

1. **Puppies (up to 1 year)**
   - Caloric Needs: 30-40 kcal per pound of body weight per day
   - Serving Size: Approx. 3-5 cups per day, divided into 3-4 meals
2. **Adults (1-7 years)**
   - Caloric Needs: 20-30 kcal per pound of body weight per day
   - Serving Size: Approx. 4-6 cups per day, divided into 2-3 meals
3. **Seniors (7+ years)**
   - Caloric Needs: 15-25 kcal per pound of body weight per day
   - Serving Size: Approx. 3-5 cups per day, divided into 2-3 meals

Medium Breed Dogs (20-50 lbs)

1. **Puppies (up to 1 year)**
   - Caloric Needs: 35-45 kcal per pound of body weight per day
   - Serving Size: Approx. 2-4 cups per day, divided into 3-4 meals
2. **Adults (1-7 years)**
   - Caloric Needs: 25-35 kcal per pound of body weight per day
   - Serving Size: Approx. 3-4 cups per day, divided into 2-3 meals
3. **Seniors (7+ years)**
   - Caloric Needs: 20-30 kcal per pound of body weight per day
   - Serving Size: Approx. 2-3 cups per day, divided into 2-3 meals

Small Breed Dogs (Up to 20 lbs)

1. **Puppies (up to 1 year)**
   - Caloric Needs: 40-50 kcal per pound of body weight per day
   - Serving Size: Approx. 1-2 cups per day, divided into 3-4 meals
2. **Adults (1-7 years)**
   - Caloric Needs: 30-40 kcal per pound of body weight per day
   - Serving Size: Approx. 1.5-2.5 cups per day, divided into 2-3 meals
3. **Seniors (7+ years)**
   - Caloric Needs: 25-35 kcal per pound of body weight per day
   - Serving Size: Approx. 1-2 cups per day, divided into 2-3 meals

REHEATING AND FREEZING TIPS

Proper reheating and freezing techniques are essential for maintaining the quality, safety, and nutritional integrity of homemade dog food. Whether you're preparing meals in advance or have leftovers to store, following these tips will help ensure that your dog's food remains safe and appetizing

Reheating Tips

1. **Thaw Safely:** If you're reheating frozen homemade dog food, thaw it safely in the refrigerator overnight or in cold water for quicker thawing. Avoid thawing at room temperature or using the microwave, as these methods can promote bacterial growth and compromise food safety.

2. **Use Gentle Heat:** When reheating homemade dog food, use gentle heat to avoid overcooking or damaging the nutrients in the food. Heat the food slowly over low to medium heat, stirring occasionally to ensure even heating.

3. **Monitor Temperature:** Use a food thermometer to monitor the temperature of reheated dog food, ensuring it reaches a safe internal temperature of 165°F (74°C) to kill any bacteria or pathogens that may be present.

4. **Avoid Overheating:** Be cautious not to overheat homemade dog food, as this can result in nutrient loss and changes in texture or taste. Remove the food from the heat source as soon as it reaches the desired temperature and allow it to cool slightly before serving.

5. **Serve Promptly:** Once reheated, serve homemade dog food promptly to prevent it from sitting at room temperature for an extended period. If there are leftovers, refrigerate or freeze them promptly to maintain freshness and safety.

Freezing Tips

1. **Divide into Portions:** Before freezing homemade dog food, divide it into individual servings or portions to make it easier to thaw and serve as needed. Use freezer-safe containers or resealable bags to store the portions, ensuring they are tightly sealed to prevent freezer burn and maintain freshness.

2. **Label and Date:** Label each container or bag with the contents and date of preparation before freezing. Proper labeling allows you to keep track of the food's freshness and ensures timely consumption.

3. **Freeze Quickly:** Freeze homemade dog food as quickly as possible after preparation to preserve its quality and nutritional value. Place the portions in the freezer promptly and spread them out in a single layer to promote rapid freezing.

4. **Avoid Overfilling:** Avoid overfilling containers or bags with homemade dog food, as this can prevent proper airflow and lead to uneven freezing. Leave some space at the top of each container or bag to allow for expansion as the food freezes.

5. **Use within Recommended Timeframe:** Follow recommended guidelines for storing frozen homemade dog food and use it within the recommended timeframe to ensure optimal quality and safety. While homemade dog food can typically be stored in the freezer for several months, it's best to consume it within a reasonable timeframe to maintain freshness and nutritional integrity.

BONUSES

To receive your free bonuses, please email me at **bluriverpublishinghouse@gmail.com**, indicating the title of the book "Slow Cooker Dog Food Cookbook" in the subject line.

CONCLUSION

———————

In this book, we've explored the collaboration of nutrition and canine well-being. Through a selection of slow cooker recipes tailored specifically for our four-legged companions, we've discovered the art of crafting wholesome meals with wholesome ingredients. We began with an understanding of the importance of balanced nutrition in maintaining optimal health for dogs, emphasizing the significance of protein, carbohydrates, fats, vitamins, and minerals in their diets. From there, we delved into the intricacies of various health conditions that dogs may encounter throughout their lives, including dental issues, obesity, ear infections, arthritis, urinary tract infections, and renal disease. With each condition, we curated recipes designed to address specific dietary needs, whether it be soft textures for dental health, low-fat options for weight management, or ingredients rich in anti-inflammatory properties to alleviate discomfort.

One thing is clear: the slow cooker is not just a kitchen appliance; it's a tool for nurturing, healing, and enhancing the lives of our beloved canine companions. From savory stews to nutrient-packed soups and casseroles, each recipe was crafted with the utmost care and attention to detail. Every dish serves a purpose beyond mere sustenance—it's a gesture of love and devotion from pet parents to fur babies.

The slow cooker offers unparalleled convenience for busy pet parents seeking to provide homemade meals without the hassle. With minimal prep time and hands-off cooking, the slow cooker becomes a time-saving ally in the quest for wholesome nutrition. It's a culinary companion that allows us to prioritize our furry friends' well-being without sacrificing our hectic schedules.

But *Slow Cooker Dog Food* is more than just a collection of recipes; it's a celebration of the bond between humans and dogs. Through the act of preparing homemade meals, we deepen this bond, strengthening the connection between pet parent and pup with every hearty meal shared.

As we conclude our culinary journey through the world of slow cooker dog food, let us carry forth the lessons learned and the recipes shared, knowing that we hold in our hands the power to nurture, heal, and uplift the lives of our furry friends. May each meal served be a reflection of our love, our dedication, and our unwavering commitment to the well-being of our canine companions. May the bond we share with our dogs continue to flourish, strengthened by the nourishment of body, mind, and soul found in every lovingly prepared dish.

Made in United States
Orlando, FL
15 September 2024

51532858R00070